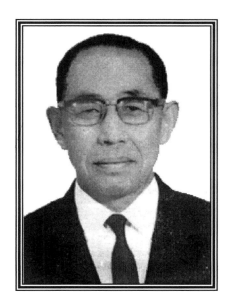

Tung Acupuncture

A Quick
Reference Guide

By:
 Theodore L. Zombolas PhD(AM), LAc, Dipl.Ac. (NCCAOM)

Forward by:
Mansoor Husain M.D., LAc.

I

Tung Acupuncture: A Quick Reference Guide

Copyright

Dedication:

To my wife Karen who put up with my absence during the research and compilation of this book, and who's support and love would not have made this book possible.

Also to my two sons Christopher and Nicholas, who have given me many reasons to improve the world, we live in.

I would like to thank James Maher for his help with completing this book. He was instrumental in guiding me through some difficult translations, as well as guidance with fine-tuning of the manuscript.

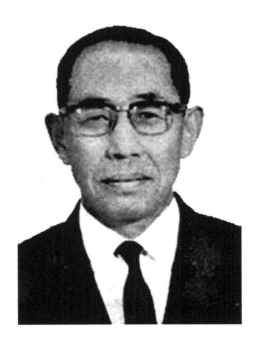

Master Tung Ching Chang
1916 – 1975

I would like to take this opportunity to first and foremost thank Master Tung Ching Chang for sharing his knowledge of acupuncture. This has ensured that his family style of acupuncture, which has survived many generations, will live on through his 73 disciples and their students.

I was very fortunate to be one of those students, studying Master Tung's Orthodox Acupuncture under Master Tung's disciple, Dr. Palden Carson. Through Dr. Carson's tutelage and direction, I have achieved "Advanced Level" in Master Tung's Orthodox Acupuncture. To this, I thank Dr. Palden Carson for his teachings, guidance and friendship, for which I have become a better acupuncturist, benefiting my patients for many years to come.

Forward

Traditional Chinese Medicine encompasses a wide range of styles and practioners that are associated with a myriad of philosophies, points, and indications. There exists a multitude of books and charts that facilitate learning this. Over the course of several hundred years, the Tung family quietly developed a style of acupuncture using predominantly the extremities and constructed their own unique point and nomenclature system. Learning this new method can be a daunting task. However, until now, there exists no compendium that organizes all the points and clinical indications that encompass Master Tung's style of acupuncture.

Ted Zombolas has filled this void with a thoroughly researched and cross-checked reference manual. This manual includes a brief background of Master Tung and his unique acupuncture school. An exhaustive list of clinical conditions which match a hierarchy of exclusive Tung's points, both individual and Dao Ma (combinations), is detailed. Particularly potent points for a given indication are highlighted and secondary points are listed underneath. Indications for micro-puncture, which Master Tung used extensively, are also included. Valuable instructions regarding location, angle and depth of needle insertion are succinctly described.

This practical manual will serve as a necessary companion to any beginning student of Tung's style acupuncture. It will be a handy reference to more experienced Tung's practitioners when dealing with less frequently seen conditions.

Ted is a gifted teacher and practitioner of the Martial Arts, Herbal Therapy, Traditional Chinese Acupuncture, and Master Tung's style acupuncture. He has put the same enthusiasm and care into this manual that he puts into his clinical practice. I commend Ted for the time and effort he has put into this work and thank him for his effort in promoting Master Tung's style of acupuncture in this country.

Mansoor Husain, M.D.
Albert Einstein Pain Institute
Clinical Director of Anesthesiology
Albert Einstein Medical Center
Assistant Professor of Anesthesiology
Thomas Jefferson University School of Medicine

Introduction:

Over the past few years, there have been a greater number of Tung style acupuncture books on the market in the English language. Most books written on this subject are in Chinese and of these, only a few have been translated or condensed onto the English language. This has afforded the non Chinese-speaking acupuncturists the ability to read and learn about this exceptional family style of acupuncture. The majority of books available today are point location style books. This is in part because Master Tung authorized the only book on his style to be published on point location with no theoretical explanation. This "cookbook" style of acupuncture differs widely to the popular traditional Chinese medicine (TCM) acupuncture of the People's Republic of China (PRC).

Although there are a number of Tung style points that are similar in location to the PRC TCM acupuncture, the indications for those points are different. The use of distal needling along with contra lateral needling allows the patient to move the affected area. This results in immediate scrutiny as to the effectiveness of the treatment. As a result the practitioner can alter the treatment plan depending on the patient's immediate feedback.

This quick reference guide was created from my personal Tung acupuncture notes including review of currently available English Tung acupuncture books on the market at the time of this writing. Some may liken it to a "Cheat Book" used to look up points, which have not been used on a routine basis that require a swift reminder on indication and likely point combinations. It is a quick reference guide that is meant to be used by practitioners who are already versed in the Tung style of acupuncture. With this in mind, point location has been deliberately omitted from this book, as knowledge of these points and locations should already be in the practitioner's repertoire. Today there are a number of Tung style acupuncture point location books on the market, which can fill the void as needed.

In the quick reference guide, you will notice bold characters on some of the indications. This indicates that this point combination for the particular indication will afford the best results based on my own experience. This may not be your experience, and therefore you are not required to follow my lead. It is merely an "at a glance" support feature. It is not meant for the practitioner to follow blindly. Individual practitioners may have their own tried and proven point combinations, which should be followed based on their own experience. You will also notice that there are more than one possible combinations of points for a similar condition, choose the point prescription that best suits your current level of training or comfort level. Properly trained practitioners versed in this style of acupuncture should constantly achieve desired results. It is strongly suggested and encouraged that practitioners wishing to learn Tung acupuncture, seek out and study with qualified teachers.

Tung style acupuncture also incorporates the method of micro-puncture routinely. A brief section on the method of micro-puncture is included for historic purposes and as a refresher, and is best applied by properly trained personnel.

Theodore Zombolas PhD (AM), LAc
2011

Who is Master Tung Ching Chang?

Tung Ching-Chang (known today as Master Tung) was born a Doaist in 1916 in the town of Ping Du County, Shandong Province of Northern China. The only heir of the now known Tung's Orthodox Acupuncture (TOA). A treasured family secret handed down from father to eldest son and refined over many generations that can be traced back 1800 years. Master Tung's family's system of Chinese Medicine incorporates bloodletting techniques along with acupuncture, very effectively. In most cases the patient notices the effect immediately upon needle insertion. Tung's Orthodox Acupuncture has approximately 500 points in all, with most used points situated on the limbs. This method has an inherent safety feature, as the possibility of organ damage by needle is non-existent, which is the case with traditional Chinese medicine (TCM) acupuncture.

Following the Communist victory on Mainland China in 1949, Master Tung, as a member of President Chang Kai Shek's Kuomintang (K.M.T.) National Army, fled to Taiwan. During this time, Master Tung gained a remarkable reputation by providing free acupuncture services to his military colleagues. Because of this, when he left the army, he was asked by his previous patients and colleagues to open his own Tung's Acupuncture practice in Taipei City.

Master Tung was an acupuncture physician in Taiwan for 26 years. Between the years of 1953-1975, he had over 400,000 patient visits with at least 100,000 at no cost in his clinic in Taipei. With strong religious beliefs and compassion towards all of his patients he never discriminated against anyone, and all were treated regardless of their ability to pay.

Master Tung started to take on apprentices and disciples in order to pass on his knowledge of his superior art of Eastern Medicine. His selection process for disciples was constantly evolving. Initially he took on students from his native Shandong province, and later from all nationalities to include Taiwan Chinese, Vietnamese and Canadian medical doctors.

He had a strict policy of whom he would accept as a student and whom he would not accept. Although many have been to his clinic and observed, only the 73 chosen disciples Master Tung took on as students, have their names engraved on his epitaph. This ensured that there were no questions as to who was and was not an accepted student of Master Tung.

In his clinic, Master Tung was a man of little words. His disciples observed and learned during the course of the day. If there were any questions, Master Tung would have the disciples try to figure out the problem for them selves, and offered guidance when necessary. The points he used are unique in that they are located opposite the affected area. This allowed the patient to move the affected area once needle insertion was complete. With this, immediate results were not only obtained, but the high effectiveness of TOA was evident. Master Tung often inserted needles through the patients clothing. This made exact location of points difficult for occasional observers to learn. Only with time and

IX

direction were disciples able to accurately locate and insert needles with the accuracy and manual dexterity of Master Tung.

With the encouragement of his current disciples, Master Tung authorized his student Yuan Kuo Pen to write down his points and indications. This book was published in Chinese for the first time in August 1973. Master Tung instructed Dr. Palden Carson to translate the book into English for the benefit of visiting doctors that could not speak or read Chinese. Dr. Carson was chosen because of his western medical background and strong commitment to Master Tung. The first English version of Master Tung's acupuncture was first published in December 1973. In 1988, Dr. Carson added his experience, re-edited and published it as "Tung's Orthodox Acupuncture". Dr. Carson chose the name of the book as Tung's Orthodox Acupuncture because it had not veered from the original teachings of Master Tung. There are no "new" points or personal interpretations of Master Tung's work by Dr. Carson in this 1988 version of the original book.

One interesting note worth mentioning is that when Master Tung was close to the end of his life, Dr. Carson visited Master Tung many times. At this time, Master Tung divulged aspects of his style of acupuncture that was not included in the original books, nor was it discussed in his clinic. This was withheld by Master Tung, and only revealed to a select few at the end. Dr. Carson took notes as Master Tung dictated over a period of time. Less than a handful of disciples that visited Master Tung in the hospital received this information.

Master Tung was famous for his wide use of Micro-puncture. Tung style micro-puncture differs from other methods as its practitioners look for most capillary dilation sites and disease referred area for bleeding purposes. Unlike other forms of bloodletting, Tung practitioners only release a few drops of blood at a time. Points over the limbs can be bled or needled, but the majority of the points on both the dorsal and ventral trunk are bled, never needled. It should be noted that micro-puncture in the hands of a poorly trained practitioner, is potentially very dangerous. Likewise, in the hands of a properly trained practitioner, the effects of micro-puncture can produce dramatic results and quicker recovery from injury. A practitioner properly trained in Tung's style acupuncture will have had proper instruction and direction in the use of micro-puncture and should be in their repertoire of techniques for treatments.

Table of Contents

Tung Acupuncture

Disease Indications
Listed
Alphabetically

Tung Acupuncture: A Quick Reference Guide

Indications	Point #	Name Pinyin	Name English	Insertion	Comments
Abdominal distension	**44.07**	**Bei Mian**	**Back Face**	**0.3-0.5 cun**	**Perpendicular insertion.**
	1010.15	**Fu Kuai**	**Bowels Ease**	**0.1-0.3 cun**	**Perpendicular insertion.**
	1010.11	Si Fu Yi	4 Bowels 1st	0.1-0.2 cun	Horizontal insertion towards 1010.10.
Abdominal distension (Cyst indigestion)	11.24	Fu Ke	Lady Class	0.2 cun	Diagonal towards index finger.
Abdominal distension (flatulence)	**88.26**	**Shang Jiu Li**	**Upper 9 Miles**	**0.8-2.0 cun**	**Perpendicular insertion.**
	1010.10	**Si Fu Er**	**4 Bowels 2nd**	**0.1-0.2 cun**	**Horizontal insertion.**
Abdominal distension Lower	22.05	Ling Gu	Androit Bone	Deep insert to 22.02	Perpendicular insertion. **Do not use on pregnant patient.**
	22.08 22.09	Wan Shun Yi Wan Shun Er	Wrist Flow One Wrist Flow Two	1.0-1.5 cun 1.0-1.5 cun	Perpendicular insertion. Add 66.05 if the pain is also on the stomach aswell.
Abdominal pain	**33.08** **33.09**	**Shou Wu Jin** **Shou Qian Jin**	**Hand Five Gold** **Hand Thousand Gold**	**0.3-0.5 cun** **0.3-0.5 cun**	**Perpendicular insertion.**
	88.04	**Jie Mei Yi**	**First Sister**	**1.5-2.0 cun**	**Perpendicular insertion.**
	1010.15	**Fu Kuai**	**Bowels Ease**	**0.1-0.3 cun**	**Perpendicular insertion.**
	11.08 **22.05** **1010.15**	**Zhi Wu Jin** **Ling Gu** **Fu Kuai**	**Finger 5 Gold** **Androit Bone** **Bowels Ease**	**0.2-0.3 cun** **Deep insert to 22.02** **0.1-0.3 cun**	**Perpendicular insertion.**
	11.08	Zhi Wu Jin	Finger 5 Gold	0.2-0.3 cun	Perpendicular insertion. Use both points.
	55.05	Hua Gu Si	Flower Bone 4	0.5-1.0 cun	Perpendicular insertion.
	66.05	Men Jin	Door Gold	0.5 cun	Perpendicular insertion Can also Micro-puncture Left for males, right for females.
Abdominal pain & distension (Lower)	22.05	Ling Gu	Androit Bone	Deep insert to 22.02	Perpendicular insertion. **Do not use on pregnant patient.**
Abdominal pain & distension (Upper)	66.05	Men Jin	Door Gold	0.5 cun	Perpendicular insertion. Very effective. For male patients use left side only, for female patiens use right side. Can also Micro-puncture
Abdominal pain lateral lower	66.05 66.11	Men Jin Hou Ju	Door Gold Fire Chrysanthemum	0.5 cun 0.5-0.8 cun	Perpendicular insertion. For male patients use left side only, for female patiens use right side. Can also Micro-puncture **Do not use 66.11on pregnant patient.**
	88.03 88.10 88.17 88.18 88.19	Tong Tian Tong Wei Zi Ma Zhong Zi Ma Shang Zi Ma Xia	Passing Sky Passing Stomach Center 4 Horses Upper 4 Horses Lower 4 Horses	0.5-1.0 cun 0.3-0.8 cun 0.8-2.5 cun 0.8-2.5 cun 0.8-2.5 cun	Perpendicular insertion.
Abdominal pain lower	33.16	Qu Ling	Curved Mound	Micro-puncture	See section on micro-puncture.
	77.09	Si Hua Zhong	4 Middle Flowers	Micro-puncture	See section on micro-puncture.
	77.09 77.14	Si Hua Zhong Si Hua Wai	4 Middle Flowers 4 Lateral Flowers	Micro-puncture	See section on micro-puncture.
Abdominal swelling (Due to flatulence)	**66.09**	**Shui Qu**	**Water Curve**	**0.5-1.0 cun**	**Perpendicular insertion.**

3

Tung Acupuncture: A Quick Reference Guide

Indications	Point #	Name Pinyin	Name English	Insertion	Comments
Abscess	**11.26**	**Zhi Wu**	**Control Dirt**	Micro-puncture	See section on micro-puncture.
	77.27	**Wai San Guan**	**Outer 3 Gates**	**1.0-1.5 cun.**	**Perpendicular insertion. Add 11.26. Similar to 5 tigers 11.27**
Acid reflux	77.17	Tian Huang	Heaven Emperor	0.5-1.0 cun	Perpendicular insertion. **Do not use 77.17 on pregnant patient.**
	77.18	Shen Guan	Kidney Gate	1.5-2.0 cun	
Acne	Ear	Back		Micro-puncture	See section on micro-puncture.
	88.17	Zi Ma Zhong	Center 4 Horses	0.8-2.5 cun	Perpendicular insertion.
	88.18	Zi Ma Shang	Upper 4 Horses	0.8-2.5 cun	
	88.19	Zi Ma Xia	Lower 4 Horses	0.8-2.5 cun	
Acne vulgaris	11.07	Zhi Si Ma	Finger 4 Horse	0.1 cun	Perpendicular insertion. Use all 3 points.
Acromion pain	22.01	Zhong Zi	Double Son	1.0-1.5 cun	Perpendicular insertion.
	22.02	Zhong Xian	Double Saint	1.0-1.5 cun	
	88.09	Tong Shen	Passing Kidney	0.3-0.5 cun	Perpendicular insertion.
	88.10	Tong Wei	Passing Stomach	0.3-0.8 cun	
	88.11	Tong Bei	Passing Back	0.5-1.0 cun	
	77.23	Ce Xia San Li	Below Lateral 3 Mile	0.5-1.0 cun	Perpendicular insertion.
	88.25	Zhong Jiu Li	Middle 9 Miles	0.8-2.0 cun	
	88.26	Shang Jiu Li	Upper 9 Miles	0.8-2.0 cun	
	88.27	Xia Jiu Li	Lower 9 Miles	0.8-2.0 cun	
Acute Cardiac rheumatism	88.01	Tong Guan	Penetrating Gate	0.3-0.5 cun	Perpendicular insertion.
	88.02	Tong Shan	Passing Mountain	0.5-0.8 cun	Only pick one or two points on one leg per treatment.
	88.03	Tong Tian	Passing Sky	0.5-1.0 cun	
Acute enteritis	77.14	Si Hua Wai	4 Lateral Flowers	1.0-1.5 cun	Perpendicular insertion.
Acute stomachache	77.09	Si Hua Zhong	4 Middle Flowers	Micro-puncture	See section on micro-puncture.
Adhesive capsulitis	**77.09**	**Si Hua Zhong**	**4 Middle Flowers**	**Micro-puncture**	**See section on micro-puncture.**
	77.10	**Si Hua Fu**	**4 Append Flowers**	**Micro-puncture**	**Right side has stronger effect.**
	88.11	Tong Bei	Passing Back	0.5-1.0 cun	Perpendicular insertion.
Albuminuria	**77.18**	**Shen Guan**	**Kidney Gate**	**1.5-2.0 cun**	**Perpendicular insertion. Highly effective**
Alcohol intoxication	**99.01**	**Er Huan**	**Ear Ring**	**0.2 cun**	**Or Micro-puncture. Insert from back to front of lobe towards root of the ear.** **Do not use with ear piercings. (Esp. hangover)**
	Ear	Tip		Micro-puncture	See section on micro-puncture.
	55.01	Huo Bao	Fire Bag	0.3-0.5 cun	Perpendicular insertion or micro-puncture. **Do not use on pregnant patient.**
Alcoholic neuritis (Pain in the hands & feet)	77.20	Si Zhi	Four Limbs	1-1.5 cun	Perpendicular insertion. Presents with slight intentional tremor. **Do not use on pregnant patient.**

Notes:

4

Tung Acupuncture: A Quick Reference Guide

Indications	Point #	Name Pinyin	Name English	Insertion	Comments
Allergic rhinitis	**88.17** **88.18** **88.19**	**Zi Ma Zhong** **Zi Ma Shang** **Zi Ma Xia**	**Center 4 Horses** **Upper 4 Horses** **Lower 4 Horses**	**0.8-2.5 cun** **0.8-2.5 cun** **0.8-2.5 cun**	**Perpendicular insertion. Treats all types of nasal diseases. Mild cases need a small number of tx. Severe cases call for more tx requiring longer retention.**
	22.14	San Cha San	Three Jam Three	1.0 – 1.5 cun	Superior point for disorders of the 5 senses. Towards the palm.
	99.05	Jin Er	Gold Ear	0.2 cun	Top ¼ of lobe.
Allergies, pollen	88.17 88.18 88.19	Zi Ma Zhong Zi Ma Shang Zi Ma Xia	Center 4 Horses Upper 4 Horses Lower 4 Horses	0.8-2.5 cun 0.8-2.5 cun 0.8-2.5 cun	Perpendicular insertion. Needle 88.17 first.
Allergies: Itching of skin due to allergies	22.14	San Cha San	Three Jam Three	1.0 – 1.5 cun	Towards the palm.
Allergy, nasal	11.17	Mu	Wood	0.25 cun	Shallow insertion, but still touch periosteum. Pinch point before insertion b/c painful.
	66.04	Hou Zhu	Fire Master	0.3-0.8 cun	Perpendicular insertion. **Do not use on pregnant patient.**
	88.17 88.18 88.19	Zi Ma Zhong Zi Ma Shang Zi Ma Xia	Center 4 Horses Upper 4 Horses Lower 4 Horses	0.8-2.5 cun 0.8-2.5 cun 0.8-2.5 cun	Perpendicular insertion.
Amenorrhea	22.05	Ling Gu	Android Bone	Deep insert to 22.02	Perpendicular insertion. Through to 22.02 bidirectional as needed. Use on any menstrual problems. **Do not use on pregnant patient.**
	66.02	Mu Fu	Wood Wife	0.2-0.4 cun	Perpendicular insertion. Use 30g-32g needle. Touch the periosteum.
	DT15	San Chiang	Three Rivers	Micro-puncture	See section on micro-puncture.
	22.05	Ling Gu	Android Bone	Deep insert to 22.02	Perpendicular insertion. **Do not use on pregnant patient.**
Anal prolapse	33.01 33.03	Qi Men Qi Zheng	This Door This Uprightness	0.2-0.5 cun 0.2-0.5 cun	Horizontal insertion. Insert in one side L or R. Can also Micro-puncture
Anemia	**77.18**	**Shen Guan**	**Kidney Gate**	**1.5-2.0 cun**	**Perpendicular insertion.**
	33.07	Huo Fu Hai	Fire Bowels	0.5-1.0 cun	Perpendicular insertion. Retain for 10 minutes, then moxa every other day for several weeks. 20 min. each time. For systemic disease do bilaterally.
Angina pectoris	**22.03**	**Shang Bai**	**Upper White**	**0.3-0.5 cun**	**Perpendicular insertion.**
	55.01	**Huo Bao**	**Fire Bag**	**0.3-0.5 cun**	**Perpendicular insertion. Micro-puncture to enhance the therapeutic effect. Do not use on pregnant patient.**
	33.14	Di Shi	Earth Scholar	1.0-1.5 cun	Perpendicular insertion.
	44.09 44.10	Di Zong Tian Zong	Earth Ancestor Heaven Ancestor	1.0-2.0 cun 1.0-1.5 cun	Perpendicular insertion. Bilateral 44.09 for better results. Add 55.01 to enhance the treatment.
	66.03 66.04	Huo Ying Huo Zhu	Fire Hardness Fire Master	0.3-0.5 cun 0.3-0.8 cun	Perpendicular insertion. Add 55.01 to enhance the treatment. **Do not use these points on pregnant patient.**

5

Tung Acupuncture: A Quick Reference Guide

Indications	Point #	Name Pinyin	Name English	Insertion	Comments
Ankle injury (External ligament)	22.06 22.07	**Zhong Bai** **Xia Bai**	**Center White** **Lower White**	**0.3-0.5 cun** **0.3-0.5 cun**	**Perpendicular insertion. Can also use 11.21, 1010.22**
Ankle pain	**11.29**	**Lau Hu**	**A Tiger**	**0.1 cun**	**Perpendicular insertion.**
	11.19 **11.29** **22.06**	**Xin Chang** **Lau Hu** **Zhong Bai**	**Heart Normal** **A Tiger** **Center White**	**0.1-0.2 cun** **0.1 cun** **0.3-0.5 cun**	**Perpendicular insertion.**
	11.27	Wu Hu	Five Tigers	0.2 cun	Perpendicular insertion. Lower body pain, ie. Feet. Use up to 3 needles
Ankle sprain	11.27	Wu Hu	Five Tigers	0.2 cun	Perpendicular insertion.
Aphasia	**88.32**	**Shi Yin**	**Voice Loss**	**1.0-1.5 cun**	**Perpendicular insertion. Keep knee at 90° angle. Micro-puncture 77.07 in severe cases.**
	1010.01	**Zheng Hui**	**Uprightness Meeting**	**0.1-0.3 cun**	**Horizontal insertion. Add 1010.08. Angle and direction of insertion is anterior to posterior insert 60°-90°.**
	1010.07	**Zong Shu**	**Total Pivot**	**0.1-0.2 cun**	**Most effective with Micro-punctureting with extreme caution. Do not exceed 0.3 cun insertion.**
Aphasia due to apoplexy	1010.20	Shui Jin	Water Gold	0.1-0.1 cun	Horizontal insertion. Bilateral.
Aphonia	88.32	Shi Yin	Voice Loss	1.0-1.5 cun	Horizontal insertion.
	1010.07	Zong Shu	Total Pivot	Micro-puncture	See section on micro-puncture.
Aphthae (Mouth ulcer)	**77.15** **77.16**	**Shang Chun** **Xia Chun**	**Upper Lip** **Lower Lip**	**Micro-puncture** **Micro-puncture**	**See section on micro-puncture. Have patient bend knees to expose points.**
Aplastic anemia	33.11	Gan Men	Liver Gate	1.0-1.5 cun	Perpendicular insertion. Insert next to the bone. **Always use left arm.** CW= releases chest tension, CCW= for intestinal pain.
	66.06 66.07	Mu Liu Mu Dou	Wood Stay Wood Scoop	0.3-0.5 cun 0.3-0.5 cun	Perpendicular insertion.
	88.12 88.13 88.14	Ming Huang Tian Huang Qi Huang	Bright Yellow Heavenly Yellow This Yellow	1.5-2.5 cun 1.5-2.5 cun 1.5-2.0 cun	Perpendicular insertion.
Appendicitis	**66.05**	**Men Jin**	**Door Gold**	**0.5 cun**	**Perpendicular insertion. Can also Micro-puncture Left for males, right for females.** **Most effective points for appendicitis.**
	77.09 77.14	Si Hua Zhong Si Hua Wai	4 Middle Flowers 4 Lateral Flowers	Micro-puncture 1.0-1.5 cun	See section on micro-puncture. Micro-puncture 77.09 first. Then perpendicular needle. Add 66.05 to produce a better effect.
Arm cramp	33.05	Huo Ling	Fire Mound	0.5-1.0 cun	Perpendicular insertion. Contralateal.

Notes:

6

Tung Acupuncture: A Quick Reference Guide

Indications	Point #	Name Pinyin	Name English	Insertion	Comments
Arm pain	**44.16** **44.17**	**Shang Qu** **Shui Yu**	**Upper Curve** **Water Cure**	**0.6-1.5 cun** **Micro-puncture**	**Perpendicular insertion. Contra lateral.** **Can also Micro-puncture. See section on micro-puncture.**
	33.15	Tian Shi	Heaven Scholar	1.0-1.5 cun	Perpendicular insertion.
	44.08	Ren Zong	Man Ancestor	Micro-puncture	See section on micro-puncture.
	88.26	Shang Jiu Li	Upper 9 Miles	0.8-2.0 cun	Perpendicular insertion.
	DT16	Huang Ho	Paired Rivers	Micro-puncture	See section on micro-puncture.
Arm pain (Forearm)	**33.04**	**Hou Chuan**	**Fire Threaded**	**0.3-0.5 cun**	**Perpendicular insertion. Add 77.20 to enhance the therapeutic effect.**
	55.03	**Hua Gu Er**	**Flower Bone 2**	**0.5-1.0cun**	**Perpendicular insertion.**
Arm pain (Upper)	**33.15** **88.26**	**Tian Shi** **Shang Jiu Li**	**Heaven Scholar** **Shang-Chiu-Li**	**1.0-1.5 cun** **0.8-2.0 cun**	**Perpendicular insertion.**
	77.09	Si Hua Zhong	4 Middle Flowers	Micro-puncture	See section on micro-puncture.
	77.22 66.08	Ce San Li Liu Wan	Lateral 3 Mile Sixth Finish	0.5-1.0 cun 0.3-0.5 cun	Perpendicular insertion. Ipsilateral, is effective. **Do not use 66.08 on COPD, bronchiectasis or asthma patients.**
	88.25 88.26 88.27	Zhong Jiu Li Shang Jiu Li Xia Jiu Li	Middle 9 Miles Upper 9 Miles Lower 9 Miles	0.8-2.0 cun 0.8-2.0 cun 0.8-2.0 cun	Perpendicular insertion.
Armpit odor	**44.12**	**Li Bai**	**Plum White**	**0.5 cun**	**Perpendicular insertion. Add DT.01.**
	DT01 DT02	Fen Chi Shang Fen Chi Sha	Upper Separation Branch Lower Separation Branch	1.0-1.5 cun 0.5-1.0 cun	Perpendicular insertion. Bilateral
Arteriosclerosis	**44.05** **44.06**	**Hou Zhi** **Jian Zhong**	**Back Branch** **Shoulder Center**	**0.3-0.7 cun** **1.0-1.5 cun**	**Perpendicular insertion. (Due to Triglicerides, cholesterol).**
	44.06 **77.09**	**Jian Zhong** **Si Hua Zhong**	**Shoulder Center** 4 Middle Flowers	**1.0-1.5 cun** **Micro-puncture**	**Perpendicular insertion.** **See section on micro-puncture.**
	77.09 **77.10**	**Si Hua Zhong** **Si Hua Fu**	**4 Middle Flowers** **4 Append Flowers**	**Micro-puncture** **Micro-puncture**	**See section on micro-puncture.** **Right side has stronger effect.**
	44.09	Di Zong	Earth Ancestor	1.0-2.0 cun	Perpendicular insertion. Recovering point. Always use both sides for better results. 1.0 cun insertion for minor issues, 2.0 cun insertion for critical conditions.
	44.13 44.14	Zhi Tong Luo Tong	Branch Through Drop Through	1.0 cun 0.6-1.0 cun	Perpendicular insertion. Insertion along medial humerus.
	DT09	Jin Lin	Gold Forest	Micro-puncture	See section on micro-puncture.
Arthralgia	**66.09**	**Shui Qu**	**Water Curve**	**0.5-1.0 cun**	**Perpendicular insertion. All joints, whole body pain, arthritis type.**
Arthritic pain of the fingers	**88.02**	**Tong Shan**	**Passing Mountain**	**0.5-0.8 cun**	**Perpendicular insertion.**
Arthritis (RA, OA)	**11.16**	**Huo Xi**	**Fire Knee**	**0.1 cun**	**Perpenducular insertion.**
Arthritis (Esp. elbow)	**33.16**	**Qu Ling**	**Curved Mound**	**0.3-0.5 cun**	**Perpendicular insertion. Contra lateral.**

7

Tung Acupuncture: A Quick Reference Guide

Indications	Point #	Name Pinyin	Name English	Insertion	Comments
Arthritis rheumatoid	77.17	Tian Huang	Heaven Emperor	0.5-1.0 cun	Perpendicular insertion. **Do not use on pregnant patient.**
Asthma (In children)	22.04	Da Bai	Big White	Deep insert to 22.01	Perpendicular insertion. Bidirectional as needed. Can also Micro-puncture **Do not use on pregnant patients.**
Asthma	**44.08**	**Ren Zong**	**Man Ancestor**	**0.5 cun**	**Perpendicular insertion. Caution Biceps muscle or Cephalic vein.**
	77.08 **77.09** **77.10**	**Si Hua Shang** **Si Hua Zhong** **Si Hua Fu**	**4 Upper Flowers** **4 Middle Flowers** **4 Append Flowers**	**2.0-3.0 cun** **2.0-3.0 cun** **Micro-punture**	**Perpendicular insertion. 28g needle. Right side has stronger effect.**
	77.14	**Si Hua Wai**	**4 Lateral Flowers**	**1.0-1.5 cun**	**Perpendicular insertion. 28g needle, or Micro-puncture**
	33.07	Huo Fu Hai	Fire Bowels	0.5-1.0 cun	Perpendicular insertion. For systemic disease do bilaterally.
	33.16	Qu Ling	Curved Mound	0.3-0.5 cun	Perpendicular insertion.
	88.17 88.18 88.19	Zi Ma Zhong Zi Ma Shang Zi Ma Xia	Center 4 Horses Upper 4 Horses Lower 4 Horses	0.8-2.5 cun 0.8-2.5 cun 0.8-2.5 cun	Perpendicular insertion.
	1010.02 1010.03 1010.04	Zhou Yuan Zhou Kun Zhou Lun	Prefecture Round Prefecture Elder Brother Prefecture Mountain	0.1-0.3 cun 0.1-0.3 cun 0.1-0.3 cun	Horizontal insertion.
	1010.19 1010.20	Shui Tong Shui Jin	Water Through Water Gold	0.1-0.5 cun 0.1-0.5 cun	Horizontal insertion. Bilateral.
Asthma (Adult) Acute or chronic	**33.13** **33.14** **33.15**	**Ren Shi** **Di Shi** **Tian Shi**	**Human Scholar** **Earth Scholar** **Heaven Scholar**	**0.5-1.0 cun** **1.0-1.5 cun** **1.0-1.5 cun**	**Perpendicular insertion. Always use 33.13, 33.14 and 33.15 together with 22.05 bilaterally. Acute = shallow insertion, Chronic = deep insertion.**
Asthma adult	VT02	Shi Er Hou	12 Monkeyes	Micro-puncture	See section on micro-puncture.
Asthmatic breathing	**1010.19** **1010.20**	**Shui Tong** **Shui Jin**	**Water Through** **Water Gold**	**0.1-0.5 cun** **0.1-0.5 cun**	**Horizontal insertion. Bilateral.**
	22.01 22.02	Zhong Zi Zhong Xian	Double Son Double Saint	1.0-1.5 cun 1.0-1.5 cun	Perpendicular insertion.
	22.04	Da Bai	Big White	Micro-puncture	See section on micro-puncture. **Do not use on pregnant patient.**
	22.11	Tu Shui	Earth Water	0.2-0.3 cun	Perpendicular insertion.
	33.16	Qu Ling	Curved Mound	Micro-puncture	See section on micro-puncture.
	77.09 77.14	Si Hua Zhong Si Hua Wai	4 Middle Flowers 4 Lateral Flowers	Micro-puncture Micro-puncture	See section on micro-puncture.
	1010.19	Shui Tong	Water Through	0.1-0.5 cun	Horizontal insertion. Bilateral.

Notes:

Tung Acupuncture: A Quick Reference Guide

Indications	Point #	Name Pinyin	Name English	Insertion	Comments
Astigmatism (Distorted vision)	**77.18**	**Shen Guan**	**Kidney Gate**	**1.5-2.0 cun**	**Perpendicular insertion.**
	77.28	**Guang Ming**	**Bright Light**	**0.5-1.0 cun**	**Perpendicular insertion. Use thinner needle 30g.**
	22.06	Zhong Bai	Center White	0.3-0.5 cun	Perpendicular insertion.
	22.06	Zhong Bai	Center White	0.3-0.5 cun	Perpendicular insertion. Can also use
	22.07	Xia Bai	Lower White	0.3-0.5 cun	11.21, 1010.22
	77.18	Shen Guan	Kidney Gate	1.5-2.0 cun	Perpendicular insertion.
	77.28	Guang Ming	Bright Light	0.5-1.0 cun	
	99.06	Shui Er	Water Ear	0.2 cun	Slightly behind Nogier's cervical spine point.
Ateriosclerosis	DT05	Shuang Feng	Double Phoenix	Micro-puncture	See section on micro-puncture.
	DT04	Wu Ling	5 Mountain Ranges	Micro-puncture	See section on micro-puncture.
	77.09	Si Hua Zhong	4 Middle Flowers	Micro-puncture	See section on micro-puncture.
	77.14	Si Hua Wai	4 Lateral Flowers		
Augment breast size	**11.14**	**Zhi San Zhong**	**Finger 3 Layer**	**0.1 cun**	**Perpenducular insertion. Use all 3 points.** **Add 77.05 to enhance the thearaputic effect**
Back & spine deformity	88.03	Tong Tian	Passing Sky	0.5-1.0 cun	Perpendicular insertion.
	88.12	Ming Huang	Bright Yellow	1.5-2.5 cun	
	88.14	Qi Huang	This Yellow	1.5-2.0 cun	
Back (Low) soreness	66.12	Huo San	Fire Scatter	0.5-1.0 cun	Horizontal insertion. **Do not use on pregnant patients.**
Back ache (Unilateral)	22.01	Zhong Zi	Double Son	1.0-1.5 cun	Perpendicular insertion.
	22.02	Zhong Xian	Double Saint	1.0-1.5 cun	
Back ache (Bilateral)	22.01	Zhong Zi	Double Son	1.0-1.5 cun	Perpendicular insertion. Needle one point on each side.
	22.02	Zhong Xian	Double Saint	1.0-1.5 cun	
	77.03	Zheng Shi	Upright Scholar	0.5-1.0 cun	Perpendicular insertion.
	77.04	Bo Qiu	Catching Ball	1.0-2.0 cun	
Back ache	88.11	Tong Bei	Passing Back	0.5-1.0 cun	Perpendicular insertion.
	88.17	Zi Ma Zhong	Center 4 Horses	0.8-2.5 cun.	Perpendicular insertion.
	88.18	Zi Ma Shang	Upper 4 Horses	0.8-2.5 cun	
	88.19	Zi Ma Xia	Lower 4 Horses	0.8-2.5 cun	
Back ache radiating to lower limb	1010.13	Ma Jin Shui	Horse Gold Water	0.1-0.3 cun	Perpendicular insertion.
Back ache to neck	22.02	Zhong Xian	Double Saint	1.0-1.5 cun	Perpendicular insertion.
Back ache to shoulder	22.01	Zhong Zi	Double Son	1.0-1.5 cun	Perpendicular insertion.

Notes:

Tung Acupuncture: A Quick Reference Guide

Indications	Point #	Name Pinyin	Name English	Insertion	Comments
Back pain	**11.15**	**Zhi Shen**	**Finger Kidney**	**0.1 cun**	**Perpenducular insertion. Use all 3 points.**
	22.04 **22.05** **22.06**	**Da Bai** **Ling Gu** **Zhong Bai**	**Big White** **Androit Bone** **Center White**	Deep insert to 22.01 Deep insert to 22.02 0.3-0.5 cun	**Perpendicular insertion.**
	33.13	**Ren Shi**	**Human Scholar**	**0.5-1.0 cun**	**Perpendicular insertion.**
	22.01	Zhong Zi	Double Son	1.0-1.5 cun	Perpendicular insertion.
	22.02	Zhong Xian	Double Saint	1.0-1.5 cun	Perpendicular insertion.
	22.06 22.07	Zhong Bai Xia Bai	Center White Lower White	0.3-0.5 cun 0.3-0.5 cun	Perpendicular insertion.
	22.08 22.09	Wan Shun Yi Wan Shun Er	Wrist Flow One Wrist Flow Two	1.0-1.5 cun 1.0-1.5 cun	Perpendicular insertion.
	55.04	Hua Gu San	Flower Bone 3	0.8 cun	Perpendicular insertion.
	66.12	Huo San	Fire Scatter	0.5-1.0 cun	Horizontal insertion. Use on one side only. Always use with 66.10 & 66.11. **Do not use on pregnant patient.**
	88.10 88.11	Tong Wei Tong Bei	Passing Stomach Passing Back	0.3-0.8 cun 0.5-1.0 cun	Perpendicular insertion.
	88.15	Huo Zhi	Fire Branch	1.5-2.0 cun	Perpendicular insertion.
	88.16	Huo Quan	Fire Complete	1.5-2.0 cun	Perpendicular insertion.
	88.17 88.18 88.19	Zi Ma Zhong Zi Ma Shang Zi Ma Xia	Center 4 Horses Upper 4 Horses Lower 4 Horses	0.8-2.5 cun. 0.8-2.5 cun 0.8-2.5 cun	Perpendicular insertion. Contralateral
	88.27	Xia Jiu Li	Lower 9 Miles	0.8-2.0 cun	Perpendicular insertion.
Back pain (Bilateral)	**22.06** **22.07** **22.08**	**Zhong Bai** **Xia Bai** **Wan Shun Yi**	**Center White** **Lower White** **Wrist Flow One**	**0.3-0.5 cun** **0.3-0.5 cun** **1.0-1.5 cun**	**Perpendicular insertion. Can also use 11.21, 1010.22**
Back pain low	**77.01** **77.02**	**Zheng Jin** **Zheng Zong**	**Upright Tendon** **Uprightness Ancestry**	**0.5-0.8 cun** **0.5-0.8 cun**	**Perpendicular insertion. Insertion through the Achilles tendon. Contra lateral insertion first, then ipsi lateral insertion. Always use 77.02 with 77.01 for better results.**
	22.14	San Cha San	Three Jam Three	1.0 – 1.5 cun	Towards the palm.
	44.13 44.14	Zhi Tong Luo Tong	Branch Through Drop Through	1 cun 0.6-1.0 cun	Perpendicular insertion. Insertion along medial humerus.
	66.14 66.15	Shui Xiang Shui Xian	Water Phase Water Fairy	0.3-0.5 cun 0.5 cun	Perpendicular insertion through anterior margin of the tendon.
Back sorness	1010.22	Bi Yi	Nasal Wing	0.1-0.2 cun	Perpendicular insertion.
Back tenderness	88.12 88.13	Ming Huang Tian Huang	Bright Yellow Heavenly Yellow	1.5-2.5 cun 1.5-2.5 cun	Perpendicular insertion.
	88.17 88.18 88.19	Zi Ma Zhong Zi Ma Shang Zi Ma Xia	Center 4 Horses Upper 4 Horses Lower 4 Horses	0.8-2.5 cun 0.8-2.5 cun 0.8-2.5 cun	Perpendicular insertion.
Backache along UB meridian	22.01 22.02	Zhong Zi Zhong Xian	Double Son Double Saint	1.0-1.5 cun 1.0-1.5 cun	Perpendicular insertion.
Bad temper	**11.17**	**Mu**	**Wood**	**0.25 cun**	**Shallow insertion, but still touch periosteum. Pinch point before insertion b/c painful.**

Notes:

10

Tung Acupuncture: A Quick Reference Guide

Indications	Point #	Name Pinyin	Name English	Insertion	Comments
Balanitis	77.18 77.19 77.21	Shen Guan Di Huang Ren Huang	Kidney Gate Earthly Emperor Man Emperor	1.5-2.0 cun 1.0-1.5 cun 0.6-1.2 cun	Perpendicular insertion. **Do not use 77.19, 77.21 on pregnant patients.**
Bed sore	**11.26**	**Zhi Wu**	**Control Dirt**	**Micro-puncture**	**See section on micro-puncture.**
Bells palsy	**11.14**	**Zhi San Zhong**	**Finger 3 Layer**	**0.1 cun**	**Perpenducular insertion. Use all 3 points.** **Add 77.28, 77.05 to enhance the thearaputic effect.**
	88.20 **88.21** **88.22**	**Xia Quan** **Zhong Quan** **Shang Quan**	**Lower Fountain** **Middle Fountain** **Upper Fountain**	**0.3-0.5 cun** **1.0-1.5 cun** **1.0-1.5 cun**	**Perpendicular insertion.**
	Ear	Apex		Micro-puncture	See section on micro-puncture.
	22.05	Ling Gu	Android Bone	Deep insert to 22.02	Perpendicular insertion. Deep insert to 22.02 bidirectional as needed. **Do not use on pregnant patient.**
Benign brain tumors	1010.04	Zhou Lun	Prefecture Mountain	0.1-0.3 cun	Horizontal insertion.
Benign laryngeal tumors	88.09 88.10 88.11	Tong Shen Tong Wei Tong Bei	Passing Kidney Passing Stomach Passing Back	0.3-0.5 cun 0.3-0.8 cun 0.5-1.0 cun	Perpendicular insertion.
Biceps tendonitis	**88.11**	**Tong Bei**	**Passing Back**	**0.5-1.0 cun**	**Perpendicular insertion.**
Biliary ascariasis	**22.06** **22.07**	**Zhong Bai** **Xia Bai**	**Center White** **Lower White**	**0.3-0.5 cun** **0.3-0.5 cun**	**Perpendicular insertion.**
Biliary colic	**22.06** **22.07**	**Zhong Bai** **Xia Bai**	**Center White** **Lower White**	**0.3-0.5 cun** **0.3-0.5 cun**	**Perpendicular insertion.**
Bladder stones	1010.13 1010.14 1010.16 1010.17	Ma Jin Shui Ma Kuai Shui Liu Kuai Qi Kuai	Horse Gold Water Horse Fast Water Six Fastness Seven Fastness	0.1-0.3 cun 0.1-0.3 cun 0.1-0.2 cun 0.5-1.5 cun	Perpendicular insertion.
Blepharitis (Eyelid inflammation)	55.02	Hua Gu Yi	Flower Bone 1	0.5-1.0 cun	Perpendicular insertion, 30g or 32g needle. Equivalent to 22.05.
Blood oozing from the wound	**11.26**	**Zhi Wu**	**Control Dirt**	**Micro-puncture**	**See section on micro-puncture.**
Blurred vision Due to hypertension	DT04	Wu Ling	5 Mountain Ranges	Micro-puncture	See section on micro-puncture. Then needle Xiasanhuang (77.17, 77.19, 77.21 **Do not use these 3 points on pregnant patient.)**

Notes:

11

Tung Acupuncture: A Quick Reference Guide

Indications	Point #	Name Pinyin	Name English	Insertion	Comments
Blurred vision	22.08 22.09	**Wan Shun Yi** Wan Shun Er	**Wrist Flow One** Wrist Flow Two	**1.0-1.5 cun** **1.0-1.5 cun**	**Perpendicular insertion. Esp. for female but only pick in one hand.**
	1010.09 1010.10 1010.11	**Shang Li** **Si Fu Er** **Si Fu Yi**	**Upper Mile** **4 Bowels 2nd** **4 Bowels 1st**	**0.1-0.2 cun** **0.1-0.2 cun** **0.1-0.2 cun**	**Horizontal insertion to 1010.01 or 1010.08.** **Insertion towards 1010.10.**
	33.10	Chang Men	Intestine Gate	1.0-1.5 cun	Perpendicular insertion. Insertion next to the bone. **Always use left arm.**
	66.11	Huo Ju	Fire Chrysanthemum	0.5-0.8 cun	Horizontal insertion. Use only one point in one treatment. **Do not use on pregnant patient.**
	66.12	Huo San	Fire Scatter	0.5-0.8 cun	Horizontal insertion. Only one point in one treatment. **Do not use on pregnant patients.**
	77.18 77.28	Shen Guan Guang Ming	Kidney Gate Bright Light	1.5-2.0 cun 0.5-1.0 cun	Perpendicular insertion.
	88.12 88.13 88.14	Ming Huang Tian Huang Qi Huang	Bright Yellow Heavenly Yellow This Yellow	1.5-2.5 cun 1.5-2.5 cun 1.5-2.0 cun	Perpendicular insertion.
	88.15	Huo Zhi	Fire Branch	1.5-2.0 cun	Perpendicular insertion.
	88.16	Huo Quan	Fire Complete	1.5-2.0 cun	Perpendicular insertion.
	99.07	Er Bei	Back of Ear	Micro-puncture	See section on micro-puncture.
Blurred vision	1010.19 1010.20	Shui Tong Shui Jin	Water Through Water Gold	0.1-0.5 cun 0.1-0.5 cun	Horizontal insertion. Bilateral.
Body odor	44.10	Tian Zong	Heaven Ancestor	1.0-1.5 cun	Perpendicular insertion. Caution to Biceps muscle or Cephalic vein.
Bone diseases	22.05 66.04	Ling Gu Huo Zhu	Androit Bone Fire Master	Deep insert to 22.02 0.3-0.8 cun	Perpendicular insertion. Insert needle along the bones. **Do not use these points on pregnant patient.**
Bone swelling in all extremities,	22.08 22.09	**Wan Shun Yi** **Wan Shun Er**	**Wrist Flow One** **Wrist Flow Two**	**1.0-1.5 cun** **1.0-1.5 cun**	**Perpendicular insertion. Esp. for female but only pick in one hand.**
Bone swelling of all body	**11.27**	**Wu Hu**	**Five Tigers**	**0.2 cun.**	**Perpendicular insertion.**
Bone swelling	**22.06** **22.07**	**Zhong Bai** **Xia Bai**	**Center White** **Lower White**	**0.3-0.5 cun** **0.3-0.5 cun**	**Perpendicular insertion. Can also use 11.21, 1010.22**
	22.14	**San Cha San**	**Three Jam Three**	**1.0 – 1.5 cun**	**Towards the palm.**
	77.09 **77.10**	**Si Hua Zhong** **Si Hua Fu**	**4 Middle Flowers** **4 Append Flowers**	**Micro-puncture** **Micro-puncture**	**See section on micro-puncture.** **Most imporGall Bladdert point for new growth of bone. Eg: OA, RA, capsulitis. Right side has stronger effect.**
	66.03	Huo Ying	Fire Hardness	0.3-0.5 cun	Perpendicular insertion. **Do not use on pregnant patients.**
	66.04	Huo Zhu	Fire Master	0.3-0.8 cun	Perpendicular insertion. No moxa. **Do not use on pregnant patients.**
Bone swelling (RA, OA, trauma induced)	88.12 88.13 88.14	Ming Huang Tian Huang Qi Huang	Bright Yellow Heavenly Yellow This Yellow	1.5-2.5 cun 1.5-2.5 cun 1.5-2.0 cun	Perpendicular insertion.

Notes:

Tung Acupuncture: A Quick Reference Guide

Indications	Point #	Name Pinyin	Name English	Insertion	Comments
Bradicardia	11.19 33.12	Xin Chang Xin Men	Heart Normal Heart Gate	0.1-0.2 cun 1.0-1.5 cun	Perpendicular insertion on 11.19, use both points. Perpendicular insertion on 33.12, close to bone only on left side.
	88.01 88.02 88.03	Tong Guan Tong Shan Tong Tian	Penetrating Gate Passing Mountain Passing Sky	0.3-0.5 cun 0.5-0.8 cun 0.5-1.0 cun	Perpendicular insertion.
Brain tumor	77.01	Zheng Jin	Upright Tendon	0.5-0.8 cun	Perpendicular insertion. Micro-punctureting at 77.07 San Zhong may produce a better result.
	77.07 1010.03 1010.04	San Zhong Zhou Kun Zhou Lun	Third Weight Prefecture Elder Brother Prefecture Mountain	1.0-2.0 cun 0.1-0.3 cun 0.1-0.3 cun	Horizontal insertion. Needle 1010.03 & 1010.04 then needle Dao Ma. Adding 55.06 Shang Liu, could enhance the effect. Micro-punctureting at 77.07 San Zhong may result in a better effect.
Breast augmentation	**11.14**	**Zhi San Zhong**	**Finger 3 Layer**	**0.1 cun**	**Perpenducular insertion. Use all 3 points.** **Add 77.05 to enhance the thearaputic effect**
	77.05 **77.06** **77.07**	**Yi Zhong** **Er Zhong** **San Zhong**	**First Weight** **Second Weight** **Third Weight**	**1.0-2.0 cun** **1.0-2.0 cun** **1.0-2.0 cun**	**Perpendicular insertion. Use all points bilaterally.** **This is a projection point of 11.14.**
	77.27	Wai San Guan	Outer 3 Gates	1.0-1.5 cun.	Perpendicular insertion. Similar to 5 tigers 11.27.
Breast cancer	**77.27**	**Wai San Guan**	**Outer 3 Gates**	**1.0-1.5 cun.**	**Perpendicular insertion. Similar to 5 tigers 11.27.**
Breast fibroadenomas (Benign tumor)	77.27	Wai San Guan	Outer 3 Gates	1.0-1.5 cun.	Perpendicular insertion. Similar to 5 tigers 11.27.
Breast pain	**88.17** **88.18** **88.19**	**Zi Ma Zhong** **Zi Ma Shang** **Zi Ma Xia**	**Center 4 Horses** **Upper 4 Horses** **Lower 4 Horses**	**0.8-2.5 cun.** **0.8-2.5 cun** **0.8-2.5 cun**	**Perpendicular insertion.**
Breast tumors	77.05 77.06 77.07	Yi Zhong Er Zhong San Zhong	First Weight Second Weight Third Weight	1.0-2.0 cun 1.0-2.0 cun 1.0-2.0 cun	Perpendicular insertion. Use all points bilaterally. Projection point of 11.14.
Breech presentation (At childbirth)	**66.04**	**Huo Zhu**	**Fire Master**	**0.3-0.8 cun**	**Perpendicular insertion. Do not use on pregnant patients except in this case.**
Bromhidrosis	**44.12**	**Li Bai**	**Plum White**	**0.5 cun**	**Perpendicular insertion.**
	44.10	Tian Zong	Heaven Ancestor	1.0-1.5 cun	Perpendicular insertion. Caution to Biceps muscle or Cephalic vein. Also add DT.01.
	DT01 DT02	Fen Chi Shang Fen Chi Sha	Upper Separation Branch Lower Separation Branch	1.0-1.5 cun 0.5-1.0 cun	Perpendicular insertion. Bilateral
Bronchial asthma (Esp. for children)	**22.01**	**Zhong Zi**	**Double Son**	**1.0-1.5cun**	**Perpendicular insertion.**

Tung Acupuncture: A Quick Reference Guide

Indications	Point #	Name Pinyin	Name English	Insertion	Comments
Bronchitis	**1010.19** **1010.20**	**Shui Tong** **Shui Jin**	**Water Through** **Water Gold**	**0.1-0.5 cun** **0.1-0.5 cun**	**Horizontal insertion. Bilateral. 1010.19 oblique and upward insertion subcuGall Bladdereously. Add 77.18 for chronic conditions.**
Bruxism	**77.11** **77.12**	**Si Hua Xia** **Fu Chang**	**4 Lower Flowers** **Bowels Intestine**	**0.5-1.0 cun** **0.5-1.0 cun**	**Perpendicular insertion.** **Use 30g-32g needle not thicker.**
Calf muscle pain	11.11	Fei Xin	Lung Heart	0.1 cun	Perpendicular insertion. Use both points.
	33.08 33.09	Shou Wu Jin Shou Qian Jin	Hand Five Gold Hand 1000 Gold	0.3-0.5 cun 0.3-0.5 cun	Perpendicular insertion.
Cardiac arrest	33.16	Qu Ling	Curved Mound	Micro-puncture	See section on micro-puncture.
	44.09	Di Zong	Earth Ancestor	1.0-2.0 cun	Perpendicular insertion.
	55.01	Huo Bao	Fire Bag	Micro-puncture	See section on micro-puncture. Results in fairly good effect. **Do not use on pregnant patient.**
	66.03 66.04	Huo Ying Huo Zhu	Fire Hardness Fire Master	0.3-0.5 cun 0.3-0.8 cun	Perpendicular insertion. **Do not use on pregnant patient.**
	77.09	Si Hua Zhong	4 Middle Flowers	Micro-puncture	See section on micro-puncture.
Cardiac arrhythmias	11.19 33.12	Xin Chang Xin Men	Heart Normal Heart Gate	0.1-0.2 cun 1.0-1.5 cun	Perpendicular insertion on 11.19, use both points. Perpendicular insertion on 33.12, close to bone only on left side.
Cardiac diseases	44.08 44.10	Ren Zong Tian Zong	Man Ancestor Heaven Ancestor	0.8 cun 1.0-1.5 cun	Perpendicular insertion. Strengthens the heart.
	66.03 66.04	Huo Ying Huo Zhu	Fire Hardness Fire Master	0.3-0.5 cun 0.3-0.8 cun	Perpendicular insertion. Strengthens the heart. **Do not use these points on pregnant patients.**
Cardiac pain	77.09 77.14	Si Hua Zhong Si Hua Wai	4 Middle Flowers 4 Lateral Flowers	Micro-puncture 1.0-1.5 cun	See section on micro-puncture. Perpendicular insertion.
	88.01 88.02 88.03	Tong Guan Tong Shan Tong Tian	Penetrating Gate Passing Mountain Passing Sky	0.3-0.5 cun 0.5-0.8 cun 0.5-1.0 cun	Perpendicular insertion.
Carditis	**33.12**	**Xin Men**	**Heart Gate**	**1.0-1.5 cun**	**Perpendicular insertion. Insert next to the bone. Always use left arm.**
	77.09 77.10	Si Hua Zhong Si Hua Fu	4 Middle Flowers 4 Append Flowers	Micro-puncture Micro-puncture	See section on micro-puncture. Right side has stronger effect.
Cataract	**66.14** **66.15**	**Shui Xiang** **Shui Xian**	**Water Phase** **Water Fairy**	**0.3-0.5 cun** **0.5 cun**	**Perpendicular insertion through anterior margin of the tendon. Macular problems Perpendicular insertion through flexor tetinaculum.**
	77.28	**Guang Ming**	**Bright Light**	**0.5-1.0 cun**	**Perpendicular insertion. Use thinner needle 30g.**
	77.18 77.19 77.21	Shen Guan Di Huang Ren Huang	Kidney Gate Earthly Emperor Man Emperor	1.5-2.0 cun 1.0-1.5 cun 0.6-1.2 cun	Perpendicular insertion. Retain needles for a longer time, in order to produce an enhanced effect. **Do not use 77.19, 77.21 on pregnant patient.**
Cerebral ischemia	88.01 88.02 88.03	Tong Guan Tong Shan Tong Tian	Penetrating Gate Passing Mountain Passing Sky	0.3-0.5 cun 0.5-0.8 cun 0.5-1.0 cun	Perpendicular insertion. Only pick one or two points on one leg per treatment.

Tung Acupuncture: A Quick Reference Guide

Indications	Point #	Name Pinyin	Name English	Insertion	Comments
Cerebral palsy	**1010.01**	**Zheng Hui**	**Uprightness Meeting**	**0.1-0.3 cun**	**Horizontal insertion. Add 1010.08. The angle and direction of insertion is from anterior to posterior insertion of 60°-90°.**
Cervical bone spurs with hand numbness	22.08 DT05	Wan Shun Yi Shuang Feng	Wrist Flow One Double Phoenix	1.0-1.5 cun Micro-puncture	See section on micro-puncture. You can alternate treatments with 22.04 & 22.05 contralateral.
Cervical neuralgia	**66.09**	**Shui Qu**	**Water Curve**	**0.5-1.0 cun**	**Perpendicular insertion.**
Cervical spine issues	**44.02**	**Hou Zhui**	**Back Vertibrae**	**0.3-0.5 cun**	**Perpendicular insertion. Use with 44.03.**
Cervical spondylosis	88.25	Zhong Jiu Li	Middle 9 Miles	0.8-2.0 cun	Perpendicular insertion. The right side is more powerful than left side.
Cervicitis	**11.06**	**Huan Chao**	**Return Nest**	**0.3 cun**	**Perpendicular insertion along bone. Either side, but not both.**
Chest & abdomen pain (Lateral)	88.17 88.18 88.19	Zi Ma Zhong Zi Ma Shang Zi Ma Xia	Center 4 Horses Upper 4 Horses Lower 4 Horses	0.8-2.5 cun. 0.8-2.5 cun 0.8-2.5 cun	Perpendicular insertion.
Chest & back pain	22.01 22.02 22.03	Zhong Zi Zhong Xian Shang Bai	Double Son Double Saint Upper White	1.0-1.5 cun 1.0-1.5 cun 0.3-0.5 cun	Perpendicular insertion. Contralateral.
	77.18	Shen Guan	Kidney Gate	1.5-2.0 cun	Perpendicular insertion.
	88.17 88.18 88.19	Zi Ma Zhong Zi Ma Shang Zi Ma Xia	Center 4 Horses Upper 4 Horses Lower 4 Horses	0.8-2.5 cun. 0.8-2.5 cun 0.8-2.5 cun	Perpendicular insertion.
Chest injury (Impact trauma)	77.09 77.14	Si Hua Zhong Si Hua Wai	4 Middle Flowers 4 Lateral Flowers	Micro-puncture 1.0-1.5 cun	See section on micro-puncture. Perpendicular insertion for 77.14. Micro-puncture in cases of severe injury or internal injury.
	88.17 88.18 88.19	Zi Ma Zhong Zi Ma Shang Zi Ma Xia	Center 4 Horses Upper 4 Horses Lower 4 Horses	0.8-2.5 cun. 0.8-2.5 cun 0.8-2.5 cun	Perpendicular insertion.
	88.28	Jie	Release Point	0.3-0.5 cun	Perpendicular insertion. For a recent injury. Use this point first.
Chest oppression	33.12	Xin Men	Heart Gate	1.0-1.5 cun	Perpendicular insertion. Insert next to the bone. **Always use left arm.**
	77.09	Si Hua Zhong	4 Middle Flowers	Micro-puncture	See section on micro-puncture.
	77.14	Si Hua Wai	4 Lateral Flowers	Micro-puncture	See section on micro-puncture.
Chest pain	**22.03**	**Shang Bai**	**Upper White**	**0.3-0.5 cun**	**Perpendicular insertion.**
	33.05 33.14 77.26	**Huo Ling Di Shi Qi Hu**	**Fire Mound Earth Scholar 7 Tigers**	**0.5-1.0 cun 1.0-1.5 cun 0.5-0.8 cun**	**Perpendicular insertion.**
	88.01 88.02	Tong Guan Tong Shan	Penetrating Gate Passing Mountain	0.3-0.5 cun 0.5-0.8 cun	Perpendicular insertion.
	1010.13	Ma Jin Shui	Horse Gold Water	0.1-0.3 cun	Perpendicular insertion. The right side is more effective than left side. Use the right side if patient is right handed.
	DT10	Ting Chu	Top Pillar	Micro-puncture	See section on micro-puncture.
Chest pain (Heart problem)	33.05 33.06	Huo Ling Huo Shan	Fire Mound Fire Mountain	0.5-1.0 cun 1.0-1.5 cun	Perpendicular insertion.

15

Tung Acupuncture: A Quick Reference Guide

Indications	Point #	Name Pinyin	Name English	Insertion	Comments
Chest pain lateral	66.05	Men Jin	Door Gold	0.5 cun	Perpendicular insertion. Also effective. For male patients use left side only, for female patiens use right side. Can also Micro-puncture
Chest pain to abdomen along Ren.	66.14	Shui Xiang	Water Phase	0.3-0.5 cun	Perpendicular insertion.
Chest stuffiness	11.05	Zhong Jian	Center Distance	0.2-0.3 cun	Insert perpendicular one side only.
	33.05	Hou Ling	Fire Mound	0.5-1.0 cun	Perpendicular insertion.
	33.06	Hou Shan	Fire Mountain	1.0-1.5 cun	Do not needle bilaterally.
	77.09	Si Hua Zhong	4 Middle Flowers	Micro-puncture	See section on micro-puncture.
	77.14	Si Hua Wai	4 Lateral Flowers		
	88.17	Zi Ma Zhong	Center 4 Horses	0.8-2.5 cun.	Perpendicular insertion.
	88.18	Zi Ma Shang	Upper 4 Horses	0.8-2.5 cun	
	88.19	Zi Ma Xia	Lower 4 Horses	0.8-2.5 cun	
Chest tension	33.11	Gan Men	Liver Gate	1.0-1.5 cun	Perpendicular insertion. Insert next to the bone. **Always use left arm.** CW= releases chest tension, CCW= for intestinal pain.
Cholecystitis (GB inflammation)	**66.07**	**Mu Dou**	**Wood Scoop**	**0.3-0.5 cun**	**Perpendicular insertion. 4F's: Fair, >40yo, Fat, Female.**
	88.14	**Qi Huang**	**This Yellow**	**1.5-2.0 cun**	**Perpendicular insertion.**
	88.15	**Huo Zhi**	**Fire Branch**	**1.5-2.0 cun**	
	88.16	**Huo Quan**	**Fire Complete**	**1.5-2.0 cun**	
	22.07	Xia Bai	Lower White	0.3-0.5 cun	Perpendicular insertion. Good for GB colic pain as well.
	66.05	Men Jin	Door Gold	0.5 cun	Perpendicular insertion. For male patients use left side only, for female patiens use right side. Can also Micro-puncture
	66.06	Mu Liu	Wood Stay	0.3-0.5 cun	Perpendicular insertion.
	88.12	Ming Huang	Bright Yellow	1.5-2.5 cun	Perpendicular insertion.
	88.14	Qi Huang	This Yellow	1.5-2.0 cun	
	88.15	Huo Zhi	Fire Branch	1.5-2.0 cun	
	88.25	Zhong Jiu Li	Middle 9 Miles	0.8-2.0 cun	Perpendicular insertion.
	88.26	Shang Jiu Li	Upper 9 Miles	0.8-2.0 cun	
	88.27	Xia Jiu Li	Lower 9 Miles	0.8-2.0 cun	
	1010.18	Mu Zhi	Wood Branch	0.1-0.3 cun	Perpendicular insertion.
Cholera	1010.07	Zong Shu	Total Pivot	0.1-0.2 cun	Insert downward. Most effective with Micro-punctureting with extreme caution. Only clinically used point.
Cholera with convulsions	77.04	Bo Qiu	Catching Ball	1.0-2.0 cun	Perpendicular insertion. Can also Micro-puncture 77.04.
	77.09	Si Hua Zhong	4 Middle Flowers	2.0-3.0 cun	
	77.14	Si Hua Wai	4 Lateral Flowers	1.0-1.5 cun	
Cholesterol	**44.05**	**Hou Zhi**	**Back Branch**	**0.3-0.7 cun**	**Perpendicular insertion.**
	44.06	**Jian Zhong**	**Shoulder Center**	**1.0-1.5 cun**	
Cholic pain due to renal stones	**22.07**	**Xia Bai**	**Lower White**	**0.3-0.5 cun**	**Perpendicular insertion.**
Cholilithiasis	1010.18	Mu Zhi	Wood Branch	0.1-0.3 cun	Perpendicular insertion. Add 22.07 or 88.25, 88.26 & 88.27 for a better therapeutic effect.

Tung Acupuncture: A Quick Reference Guide

Indications	Point #	Name Pinyin	Name English	Insertion	Comments
Chorea (CNS problem) (Parkinsonism)	**88.12** **88.13** **88.14**	**Ming Huang** **Tian Huang** **Qi Huang**	**Bright Yellow** **Heavenly Yellow** **This Yellow**	**1.5-2.5 cun** **1.5-2.5 cun** **1.5-2.0 cun**	**Perpendicular insertion. Add Kidney gate point 77.18. (With 77.18 total 8 points).**
Chronic Bronchitis	11.02	Xiao Jian	Small Distance	0.2-0.3 cun	Perpendicular insertion. Apply to right side.
Chronic diseases	**88.12**	**Ming Huang**	**Bright Yellow**	**1.5-2.5 cun**	**Perpendicular insertion. Insertion bi lateral.**
Chronic Fatigue	33.07	Huo Fu Hai	Fire Bowels	0.5-1.0 cun.	Perpendicular insertion. For systemic disease, do bilaterally.
Chronic fatigue (Liver deficiency) Chorea,	88.12 88.13 88.14	Ming Huang Tian Huang Qi Huang	Bright Yellow Heavenly Yellow This Yellow	1.5-2.5 cun 1.5-2.5 cun 1.5-2.0 cun	Perpendicular insertion.
Chronic fatigue (Thyroid issues)	88.18	Zi Ma Shang	Upper 4 Horses	0.8-2.5 cun	Perpendicular insertion.
Chronic fatigue Due to Kidney deficiency	1010.19 1010.20	Shui Tong Shui Jin	Water Through Water Gold	0.1-0.5 cun 0.1-0.5 cun	Horizontal insertion. Bilateral.
Chronic pain (Any type)	**1010.01** **1010.08**	**Zheng Hui** **Zhen Jing**	**Uprightness Meeting** **Tranquility**	**0.1-0.3 cun** **0.1-0.2 cun**	**Horizontal insertion.**
Chronic sinusitis	77.14	Si Hua Wai	4 Lateral Flowers	1.0-1.5 cun	Perpendicular insertion. 28g needle or Micro-puncture
Cirrhosis	44.16	Shang Qu	Upper Curve	Micro-puncture	See section on micro-puncture.
	66.06 66.07	Mu Liu Mu Dou	Wood Stay Wood Scoop	0.3-0.5 cun 0.3-0.5 cun	Perpendicular insertion.
	77.09 88.12 88.13 88.14 66.06 66.07	Si Hua Zhong Ming Huang Tian Huang Qi Huang Mu Liu Mu Dou	4 Middle Flowers Bright Yellow Heavenly Yellow This Yellow Wood Stay Wood Scoop	Micro-puncture 1.5-2.5 cun 1.5-2.5 cun 1.5-2.0 cun 1.5-2.5 cun 1.5-2.5 cun	See section on micro-puncture. Then perpendicular needle 88.12, 88.13 & 88.14 or needle 66.06 & 66.07.
Clavicle pain (Frontal)	**66.09** **77.26**	**Shui Qu** **Qi Hu**	**Water Curve** **Seven Tigers**	**0.5-1.0 cun** **0.5-0.8 cun**	**Perpendicular insertion. Use all 3 points of 77.26 at same time contra lateral.**
Cloudiness thinking and fatigue (Neurasthenia)	77.18 77.19 77.21	Shen Guan Di Huang Ren Huang	Kidney Gate Earthly Emperor Man Emperor	1.5-2.0 cun 1.0-1.5 cun 0.6-1.2 cun	Perpendicular insertion. **Do not use 77.19, 77.21 on pregnant patients.**
	1010.01 1010.08	Zheng Hui Zhen Jing	Uprightness Meeting Tranquility	0.1-0.3 cun 0.1-0.2 cun	Horizontal insertion. Micro-puncture 77.07 San Zhong after needling.
Coccyx pain	**33.12**	**Xin Men**	**Heart Gate**	**1.0-1.5 cun**	**Perpendicular insertion. Insert next to the bone. Always use left arm.**
	66.01	Hai Bao	Seal	0.1-0.3 cun	Insert 66.01 perpendicularly and contralateral.
	1010.01 1010.06	Zheng Hui Hou Hui	Uprightness Meeting Posterior Meetings	0.1-0.3 cun 0.1-0.3 cun	Horizontal insertion. 1010.06 downward insertion.
Cold sore	**77.15** **77.16**	**Shang Chun** **Xia Chun**	**Upper Lip** **Lower Lip**	**Micro-puncture** **Micro-puncture**	**See section on micro-puncture. Have patient bend knees to expose point. Lack of Vit. B-2 complex.**

17

Tung Acupuncture: A Quick Reference Guide

Indications	Point #	Name Pinyin	Name English	Insertion	Comments
Colic abdominal pain	VT05	Fu Chao 23	Bowel Nest 23	Micro-puncture	See section on micro-puncture. Not all points, but the ones closest to the umbilicus.
	77.09 77.14	Si Hua Zhong Si Hua Wai	4 Middle Flowers 4 Lateral Flowers	Micro-puncture Micro-puncture	See section on micro-puncture. Also good for abdominal colic pain.
Colitis (LI)	33.10	Chang Men	Intestine Gate	1.0-1.5 cun	Perpendicular insertion. Insertion next to the bone. **Always use left arm.**
Coma	66.03 66.04	Huo Ying Huo Zhu	Fire Hardness Fire Master	0.3-0.5 cun 0.3-0.8 cun	Perpendicular insertion. **Do not use on pregnant patients.**
	66.03 1010.01 1010.05 DT04	Huo Ying Zheng Hui Qian Hui Wu Ling	Fire Hardness Uprightness Meeting Anterior Meeting 5 Mountain Ranges	Micro-puncture 0.1-0.3 cun 0.1-0.3 cun Micro-puncture	See section on micro-puncture. Perpendicular insertion. For unconciousness Combine with 1010.08. **Do not use 66.03 on pregnant patients.**
	22.05 1010.01 1010.05 1010.06	Ling Gu Zheng Hui Qian Hui Hou Hui	Android Bone Uprightness Meeting Anterior Meeting Posterior Meetings	Deep insert to 22.02 0.1-0.3 cun 0.1-0.3 cun 0.1-0.3 cun	Horizontal insertion. **Do not use 22.05 on pregnant patient.**

Notes:

© **Theodore L. Zombolas PhD (AM), LAc, Dipl.Ac. (NCCAOM).** ©

Tung Acupuncture: A Quick Reference Guide

Indications	Point #	Name Pinyin	Name English	Insertion	Comments
Common cold	11.17	Mu	Wood	0.25 cun	Shallow insertion, but still touch periosteum. Pinch point before insertion b/c painful.
	99.08	Er San	Ear Three	Micro-puncture	See section on micro-puncture. Do bilaterally. If your treatments for common cold do not work, then Micro-puncture this point.
	33.14 33.15	Di Shi Tian Shi	Earth Scholar Heaven Scholar	1.0-1.5 cun. 1.0-1.5 cun	Perpendicular insertion. Bilateral
	44.01	Fen Jin	Dividing Gold	0.5-1.0 cun	Perpendicular insertion.
	44.08	Ren Zong	Man Ancestor	0.5 cun	Perpendicular insertion. Caution Biceps muscle or Cephalic vein.
	88.07 88.08	Gan Mao Yi Gan Mao Er	1st Catch Cold 2nd Catch Cold	0.8-1.5 cun 0.8-1.5 cun	Perpendicular insertion. Oblique insertion with 88.08. (with no muscle pain)
	Ear	Apex		Micro-puncture	See section on micro-puncture.
	DT12	Kan Mao San	3rd Catch Cold	Micro-puncture	See section on micro-puncture.
	DT04	Wu Ling	5 Mountain Ranges	Micro-puncture	See section on micro-puncture. To alleviate fever
	VT02	Shi Er Hou	12 Monkeyes	Micro-puncture	See section on micro-puncture.
	11.17 66.05	Mu Men Jin	Wood Door Gold	0.25 cun 0.5 cun	Shallow insertion for 11.17, but still touch periosteum. Pinch point before insertion b/c painful. For 66.05: For male patients use left side only, for female patiens use right side. Can also Micro-puncture
	22.01	Zhong Zi	Double Son	1.0-1.5 cun	Perpendicular insertion.
	22.14	San Cha San	Three Jam Three	1.0 – 1.5 cun	Effective for eye dryness & lacrimation due to wind. Towards the palm. Add 22.04 for headache. Add 11.17 for running nose & nasal obstruction.
	33.07	Huo Fu Hai	Fire Bowels	0.5-1.0 cun	Perpendicular insertion. For systemic disease do bilaterally.
	77.22	Ce San Li	Lateral 3 Mile	0.5-1.0 cun	Perpendicular insertion. For nasal obstruction
Common cold children	DT03	Chi Shing	Seven Stars	Micro-puncture	See section on micro-puncture. Also good with headache.
Common cold (Feverish conditions)	1010.12	Zheng Ben	Upright Source	Micro-puncture	See section on micro-puncture. Caution when Micro-punctureting not to damage the nasal cartilage.
Compartment syndrome	1010.06	Hou Hui	Posterior Meetings	0.1-0.3 cun	Insertion downward.

Notes:

19

Tung Acupuncture: A Quick Reference Guide

Indications	Point #	Name Pinyin	Name English	Insertion	Comments
Conjunctivitis (Redness of the eyes)	**22.03**	**Shang Bai**	**Upper White**	**0.3-0.5 cun**	**Perpendicular insertion.**
	55.02	**Hua Gu Yi**	**Flower Bone 1**	**0.5-1.0 cun**	**30g or 32g needle. Equivalent to 22.05.**
	66.01	**Hai Bao**	**Seal**	**0.1-0.3 cun**	**Perpendicular insertion. Contra lateral. Similar to 22.08, 22.09.**
	Ear	Apex		Micro-puncture	Very effective. See section on micro-puncture.
	66.12	Huo San	Fire Scatter	0.5-1.0 cun	Horizontal insertion. Use on one side only. Always use with 66.10 & 66.11. **Do not use on pregnant patient.**
	88.17	Zi Ma Zhong	Center 4 Horses	0.8-2.5 cun.	Perpendicular insertion.
	88.18	Zi Ma Shang	Upper 4 Horses	0.8-2.5 cun	
	88.19	Zi Ma Xia	Lower 4 Horses	0.8-2.5 cun	
Constipation	33.04	Hou Chuan	Fire Threaded	0.3-0.5 cun	Perpendicular insertion.
	L1	Shui Chung	Water Center	0.8-1.0 cun	Perpendicular insertion.
	L2	Shui Fu	Water Bowels	0.8-1.0 cun	
Contact dermatitis of hands	**11.17**	**Mu**	**Wood**	**0.25 cun**	**Shallow insertion, but still touch periosteum. Pinch point before insertion b/c painful.**
COPD Atelectasis.	22.01	Zhong Zi	Double Son	1.0-1.5 cun	Perpendicular insertion.
Coronary artery disease	DT06	Chiu Hou	9 Monkeys	Micro-puncture	See section on micro-puncture.
	11.01	Da Jian	Big Distance	0.2-0.3 cun	Perpendicular insertion. Apply to right side.
	44.09	Di Zong	Earth Ancestor	1.0-2.0 cun	Perpendicular insertion. Recovering point. Always use both sides for better results. 1.0 cun insertion for minor issues, 2.0 cun insertion for critical conditions.
	77.08	Si Hua Shang	4 Upper Flowers	3.0-3.5 cun	Perpendicular insertion.
	77.13	Si Hua Li	4 Inner Flowers	1.5-2.0 cun	Perpendicular insertion.
	88.01	Tong Guan	Penetrating Gate	0.3-0.5 cun	Perpendicular insertion.
	88.02	Tong Shan	Passing Mountain	0.5-0.8 cun	Only pick one or two points on one
	88.03	Tong Tian	Passing Sky	0.5-1.0 cun	leg per treatment.
Cosmetic	77.05	Yi Zhong	First Weight	1.0-2.0 cun	Perpendicular insertion. Clinically tend to use the right side. In males = increases pectoralis muscle. In females = increases fat tissue. Projection point of 11.14.
Costalgia (Right side in females)	**77.05**	**Yi Zhong**	**First Weight**	**1.0-2.0 cun**	**Perpendicular insertion. Use all points bilaterally.**
	77.06	**Er Zhong**	**Second Weight**	**1.0-2.0 cun**	
	77.07	**San Zhong**	**Third Weight**	**1.0-2.0 cun**	
Costalgia (Rib pain)	88.17	Zi Ma Zhong	Center 4 Horses	0.8-2.5 cun.	Perpendicular insertion. Contralateral
	88.18	Zi Ma Shang	Upper 4 Horses	0.8-2.5 cun	
	88.19	Zi Ma Xia	Lower 4 Horses	0.8-2.5 cun	
	VT03	King Wu	Gold Five	Micro-puncture	See section on micro-puncture. (Mostly due to infection).
Cough	33.07	Huo Fu Hai	Fire Bowels	0.5-1.0 cun	For systemic disease do bilaterally.
	1010.19	Shui Tong	Water Through	0.1-0.5 cun	Horizontal insertion. Bilateral.
	1010.20	Shui Jin	Water Gold	0.1-0.5 cun	

Tung Acupuncture: A Quick Reference Guide

Indications	Point #	Name Pinyin	Name English	Insertion	Comments
Cough & asthma	1010.19 1010.20	Shui Tong Shui Jin	Water Through Water Gold	0.1-0.5 cun 0.1-0.5 cun	Horizontal insertion. Bilateral.
	22.01	Zhong Zi	Double Son	1.0-1.5 cun	Perpendicular insertion. (Most effective with children)
Cramp of the foot	33.11	Gan Men	Liver Gate	1.0-1.5 cun	Perpendicular insertion. Insert next to the bone. **Always use left arm.** CW= releases chest tension, CCW= for intestinal pain.
	77.01	Zheng Jin	Upright Tendon	0.5-0.8 cun	Perpendicular insertion.
Cramp, leg	77.04	Bo Qiu	Catching Ball	1-2 cun	Perpendicular insertion. Add 77.09. (Image popleteal – scapula).
Cramping Of the hand and arm	33.06	Hou Shan	Fire Mountain	1.0-1.5 cun	Perpendicular insertion, contralateral.
Cranial bone Enlargement	77.01	Zheng Jin	Upright Tendon	0.5-0.8 cun	Perpendicular insertion. Adding 55.06 Shang Liu will produce a better result. Micro-punctureting at 77.07 San Zhong may produce a better result.
Cranial nerve Neuralgia	55.06	Shang Liu	Upper Tumor	0.3-0.5 cun	Perpendicular insertion. Deep insertion may result in dyspnea & discomfort.
Cranial tumors All types	**55.06**	**Shang Liu**	**Upper Tumor**	**0.3-0.5 cun**	**Perpendicular insertion. Deep insertion may result in dyspnea & discomfort.**
CVA	**88.29** **88.30** **88.31**	**Nei Tong Guan** **Nei Tong Shan** **Nei Tong Tian**	**Inner Passing Gate** **Inner Passing Mountain** **Inner Passing Sky**	**1.0 cun** **1.0 cun** **1.0 cun**	**Perpendicular insertion.**
	1010.06	Hou Hui	Posterior Meetings	0.1-0.3 cun	Insertion downward.
Cystitis	1010.14	Ma Kuai Shui	Horse Fast Water	0.1-0.3 cun	Perpendicular insertion.
Cystolithiasis	1010.14	Ma Kuai Shui	Horse Fast Water	0.1-0.3 cun	Perpendicular insertion.
	L2	Shui Fu	Water Bowels	0.8-1.0 cun	Perpendicular insertion.
Deafness	**55.02**	**Hua Gu Yi**	**Flower Bone 1**	**0.5-1.0 cun**	**Perpendicular insertion, 30g or 32g needle. Equivalent to 22.05.**
Delayed bone healing	**11.26**	**Zhi Wu**	**Control Dirt**	**Micro-puncture**	**See section on micro-puncture.**
Delayed wound healing	**11.26**	**Zhi Wu**	**Control Dirt**	**Micro-puncture**	**See section on micro-puncture.**
	44.05	**Hou Zhi**	**Back Branch**	**0.3-0.7 cun**	**Perpendicular insertion.**
Dermatitis, contact	11.07	Zhi Si Ma	Finger 4 Horse	0.1 cun	Perpendicular insertion. Use all 3 points.

Notes:

21

Tung Acupuncture: A Quick Reference Guide

Indications	Point #	Name Pinyin	Name English	Insertion	Comments
Diabetes mellitus	**77.17** **77.19** **77.21**	**Tian Huang** **Di Huang** **Ren Huang**	**Heaven Emperor** **Earthly Emperor** **Man Emperor**	**0.5-1.0 cun** **1.0-1.5 cun** **0.6-1.2 cun**	**Perpendicular insertion.** **Do not use these points on pregnant patient.**
	77.18	**Shen Guan**	**Kidney Gate**	**1.5-2.0 cun**	**Perpendicular insertion.**
	44.10	Tian Zong	Heaven Ancestor	1.0-1.5 cun	Perpendicular insertion. Caution Biceps muscle or Cephalic vein.
	77.17	Tian Huang	Heaven Emperor	0.5-1.0 cun	Perpendicular insertion. **Do not use on pregnant patient.**
	77.18 77.19 77.21	Shen Guan Di Huang Ren Huang	Kidney Gate Earthly Emperor Man Emperor	1.5-2.0 cun 1.0-1.5 cun 0.6-1.2 cun	Perpendicular insertion. Add 88.09 and 77.17 if thirst is present. **Do not use 77.19, 77.21 on pregnant patients.**
	77.20	Si Zhi	Four Limbs	1.0-1.5 cun	Perpendicular insertion. **Do not use on pregnant patient.**
	88.09 88.10 88.11	Tong Shen Tong Wei Tong Bei	Passing Kidney Passing Stomach Passing Back	0.3-0.5 cun 0.3-0.8 cun 0.5-1.0 cun	Perpendicular insertion. Pick 2 of these 3 points (4 points at 2 thighs), Never use 3 needles same time
	99.04	Tu Er	Earth Ear	0.2 cun	
	DT01 DT02	Fen Chi Shang Fen Chi Sha	Upper Separation Branch Lower Separation Branch	1.0-1.5 cun 0.5-1.0 cun	Perpendicular insertion. Bilateral. Use with 3 yellow points
	L2	Shui Fu	Water Bowels	0.8-1.0 cun	Perpendicular insertion.
Diarrhea acute (Imodium point)	**66.05**	**Men Jin**	**Door Gold**	**0.5 cun**	**Perpendicular insertion. Can also Micro-puncture Left for males, right for females. Can add 22.05.**
	99.08	Er San	Ear Three	Micro-puncture	See section on micro-puncture. Do bilaterally. Add 66.05.
	33.10	Chang Men	Intestine Gate	1.0-1.5 cun	Perpendicular insertion. Insertion next to the bone. **Always use left arm.**
	77.09 77.14	Si Hua Zhong Si Hua Wai	4 Middle Flowers 4 Lateral Flowers	Micro-puncture Micro-puncture	See section on micro-puncture.
Difficult delivery	22.05	Ling Gu	Androit Bone	Deep insert to 22.02	Perpendicular insertion. Deep insert to 22.02. **Do not use on pregnant patient.**
	66.04	Huo Zhu	Fire Master	0.3-0.8 cun	Perpendicular insertion. No moxa. **Do not use on pregnant patient.**
Difficult miscellaneous disease	88.25	Zhong Jiu Li	Middle 9 Miles	0.8-2.0 cun	Perpendicular insertion. Start with this point to alleviate pain, and then seek cause of disease.
Diplopia (Double vision)	**77.28**	**Guang Ming**	**Bright Light**	**0.5-1.0 cun**	**Perpendicular insertion. Use thinner needle 30g. Add 77.18 as accessory point.**
Disc problems (Severe case)	**77.10** **77.11** **77.12**	**Si Hua Fu** **Si Hua Xia** **Fu Chang**	**4 Append Flowers** **4 Lower Flowers** **Bowels Intestine**	Micro-puncture 0.5-1.0 cun 0.5-1.0 cun	**See section on micro-puncture. Perpendicular insertion. Use 30g-32g needle not thicker. Add 22.05 to enhance th therapeutic effect.**

Tung Acupuncture: A Quick Reference Guide

Indications	Point #	Name Pinyin	Name English	Insertion	Comments
Disc prolapse	**44.02**	**Hou Zhui**	**Back Vertibrae**	**0.3-0.5 cun**	**Perpendicular insertion.**
	44.03	**Shou Ying**	**Head Wisdom**	**0.3-0.5 cun**	
Disphagia Due to stroke	1010.07	Zong Shu	Total Pivot	0.1-0.2 cun	Do not exceed 0.3 cun.
Distension of the lower abdomen	11.24	Fu Ke	Lady Class	0.2 cun	Diagonal towards index finger.
Dizziness	**22.06**	**Zhong Bai**	**Center White**	**0.3-0.5 cun**	**Perpendicular insertion. Can also use 11.21, 1010.22**
	22.07	Xia Bai	Lower White	0.3-0.5 cun	
	44.13	**Zhi Tong**	**Branch Through**	**1 cun**	**Perpendicular insertion.**
	44.14	**Luo Tong**	**Drop Through**	**0.6-1.0 cun**	**Insertion along medial humerus.**
	88.01	**Tong Guan**	**Penetrating Gate**	**0.3-0.5 cun**	**Perpendicular insertion.**
	88.02	**Tong Shan**	**Passing Mountain**	**0.5-0.8 cun**	
	88.03	**Tong Tian**	**Passing Sky**	**0.5-1.0 cun**	
	11.05	Zhong Jian	Center Distance	0.2-0.3 cun	Insert perpendicular one side only.
	33.10	Chang Men	Intestine Gate	1.0-1.5 cun	Perpendicular insertion. Insertion next to the bone. **Always use left arm.**
	44.04	Fu Ding	Wealth Summit	0.5 cun	Perpendicular insertion.
	44.05	Hou Zhi	Back Branch	0.3-0.7 cun	
	66.03	Huo Ying	Fire Hardness	0.5-0.8 cun	Perpendicular insertion. **Do not use on pregnant patient.**
	66.10	Huo Lian	Fire Connection	0.5-0.8 cun	Horizontal insertion. Use on one side only. (Due to HTN). **Do not use these points on pregnant patient.**
	66.11	Huo Ju	Fire Chrysanthemum	0.5-0.8 cun	
	66.12	Huo San	Fire Scatter	0.5-1.0 cun	
	77.08	Si Hua Shang	4 Upper Flowers	3.0-3.5 cun	Perpendicular insertion.
	77.21	Ren Huang	Man Emperor	0.6-1.2 cun	Perpendicular insertion. **Do not use on pregnant patient.**
	88.15	Huo Zhi	Fire Branch	1.5-2.0 cun	Perpendicular insertion.
	88.16	Huo Quan	Fire Complete	1.5-2.0 cun	
	88.25	Zhong Jiu Li	Middle 9 Miles	0.8-2.0 cun	Perpendicular insertion. Right side is more powerful than left side.
	1010.05	Qian Hui	Anterior Meeting	0.1-0.3 cun	Insertion anterior to posterior.
	1010.06	Hou Hui	Posterior Meetings	0.1-0.3 cun	Insertion downward.
	1010.19	Shui Tong	Water Through	0.1-0.5 cun	Horizontal insertion. Bilateral. Needle to the lateral side of chin. Add 77.18 to balance Kidney Y-Y. Bilaterally.
	1010.20	Shiu Jin	Water Gold	0.1-0.5 cun	
	DT17	Chong Xiao	Expanding Heaven	Micro-puncture	See section on micro-puncture.
Double vision (Strabismus)	**77.28**	**Guang Ming**	**Bright Light**	**0.5-1.0 cun**	**Perpendicular insertion. Use thinner needle 30g. Add 77.18 as accessory point.**
	88.12	Ming Huang	Bright Yellow	1.5-2.5 cun	Perpendicular insertion.
Drooping of eye lid (Ptosis)	**77.28**	**Guang Ming**	**Bright Light**	**0.5-1.0 cun**	**Perpendicular insertion. Use thinner needle 30g. Eyes open in 3 sessions.**
Drug poisoning (Mild case)	DT01	Fen Chi Shang	Upper Separation Branch	1.0-1.5 cun	Perpendicular insertion. Bilateral
	DT02	Fen Chi Sha	Lower Separation Branch	0.5-1.0 cun	

Tung Acupuncture: A Quick Reference Guide

Indications	Point #	Name Pinyin	Name English	Insertion	Comments
Dry eyes	**11.17**	**Mu**	**Wood**	**0.25 cun**	**Shallow insertion, but still touch periosteum. Pinch point before insertion b/c painful.**
	88.12	Ming Huang	Bright Yellow	1.5-2.5 cun	Perpendicular insertion.
Dry mouth	**11.15**	**Zhi Shen**	**Finger Kidney**	**0.1 cun**	**Perpenducular insertion. Use all 3 points.**
	99.06	**Shui Er**	**Water Ear**	**0.2 cun**	
Dryness of the nose	11.17	Mu	Wood	0.25 cun	Shallow insertion, but still touch periosteum. Pinch point before insertion b/c painful. Include LI 20 to enhance the effect.
	88.17 88.18 88.19	Zi Ma Zhong Zi Ma Shang Zi Ma Xia	Center 4 Horses Upper 4 Horses Lower 4 Horses	0.8-2.5 cun 0.8-2.5 cun 0.8-2.5 cun	**Perpendicular insertion. Can treat all types of nasal diseases.**
Duodenal ulcer	22.11	**Tu Shui**	**Earth Water**	**0.2-0.3 cun**	**Perpendicular insertion.**
Dysentery	66.05	Men Jin	Door Gold	0.5 cun	Perpendicular insertion. Can also Micro-puncture. Left for males, right for females.
Dysmenorrhea	**11.06**	**Huan Chao**	**Return Nest**	**0.3 cun**	**Vertical insertion along bone. Either side, but not both.**
	11.24	**Fu Ke**	**Lady Class**	**0.2 cun**	**Diagonal towards index finger.**
	66.02	Mu Fu	Wood Wife	0.2-0.4 cun	Perpendicular insertion. Use 30g-32g needle. Touch periosteum.
	66.05	Men Jin	Door Gold	0.5 cun	Perpendicular insertion. For male patients use left side only, for female patiens use right side. Can also Micro-puncture
Dyspepsia (Indigestion)	**88.23** **88.24**	**Jin Qian Xia** **Jin Qian Shang**	**Lower Gold Front** **Upper Gold Front**	**0.3-0.5 cun** **0.5-1.0 cun**	**Perpendicular insertion.**
Dyspnoea	**77.11** **77.12**	**Si Hua Xia** **Fu Chang**	**4 Lower Flowers** **Bowels Intestine**	**0.5-1.0 cun** **0.5-1.0 cun**	**Perpendicular insertion. Use 30g-32g needle not thicker.**
	VT03	King Wu	Gold Five	Micro-puncture	See section on micro-puncture.
	11.02	Xiao Jian	Small Distance	0.2-0.3 cun	Perpendicular insertion. Apply to right side.
	33.07	Huo Fu Hai	Fire Bowels	0.5-1.0 cun	Perpendicular insertion. For systemic disease do bilaterally.
	33.15	Tian Shi	Heaven Scholar	1.0-1.5 cun	Perpendicular insertion.
	1010.19 1010.20	Shui Tong Shiu Jin	Water Through Water Gold	0.1-0.5 cun 0.1-0.5 cun	Horizontal insertion. Bilateral. Needle to the lateral side of chin. Add 77.18 to balance Kidney Y-Y. Bilaterally.
Dyspnoea, palpitations	99.03	Huo Er	Fire Ear	0.2 cun	

Notes:

24

Tung Acupuncture: A Quick Reference Guide

Indications	Point #	Name Pinyin	Name English	Insertion	Comments
Dysuria	**77.08** **88.13**	**Si Huan Shang** **Tian Huang**	**4 Upper Flowers** **Heavenly Yellow**	**2.0-3.0 cun** **1.5-2.5 cun**	**Perpendicular insertion.**
	44.06 44.11 44.15	Jian Zhong Yun Bai Xia Qu	Shoulder Center Cloud White Lower Curve	1.0-1.5 cun	Perpendicular insertion.
	66.03 66.04	Huo Ying Huo Zhu	Fire Hardness Fire Master	0.3-0.5 cun 0.3-0.8 cun	All good points for treatment. **Do not use on pregnant patients.**
	77.08 77.17	Si Hua Shang Tian Huang	4 Upper Flowers Heaven Emperor	2.0-3.0 cun 0.5-1.0 cun	Perpendicular insertion. Add 66.03 & 66.04 to enhance the therapeutic effect. **Do not use 77.17 on pregnant patients.**
	77.18 77.19 77.21	Shen Guan Di Huang Ren Huang	Kidney Gate Earthly Emperor Man Emperor	1.5-2.0 cun 1.0-1.5 cun 0.6-1.2 cun	Perpendicular insertion. **Do not use 77.19, 77.21 on pregnant patients.**
	L2	Shui Fu	Water Bowels	0.8-1.0 cun	Due to cyctitis. Perpendicular insertion.
Dysuria due to prostatitis	77.08 77.17	Si Huan Sang Tian Huang	4 Upper Flowers Heaven Emperor	2.0-3.0 cun 0.5-1.0 cun	These points will provide exceptional results. Add 66.04 along the bone to enhance the therapeutic effect. **Do not use 77.17 on pregnant patients.**
Ear distension	22.06 33.16	Zhong Bai Qu Ling	Center White Curved Mound	0.3-0.5 cun 0.3-0.5 cun	Perpendicular insertion.
Ear infection	77.14	**Si Hua Wai**	**4 Lateral Flowers**	**1.0-1.5 cun**	**Perpendicular insertion.** **28g needle or Micro-puncture**
Ear pain	77.14	Si Hua Wai	4 Lateral Flowers	1.0-1.5 cun	Perpendicular insertion. 28g needle or Micro-puncture
Ear pain (Middle ear infect)	**88.17**	**Zi Ma Zhong**	**Center 4 Horses**	**0.8-2.5 cun**	**Perpendicular insertion.**
Earache	22.14	San Cha San	Three Jam Three	1.0 – 1.5 cun	Towards the palm.
	77.07 77.14	San Zhong Si Hua Wai	Third Weight 4 Lateral Flowers	1.0-2.0 cun 1.0-1.5 cun	Perpendicular insertion. Needle simulGall Bladdereously. If prolonged, or needling is not sufficient, Micro-puncture
	77.22 77.23	Ce San Li Ce Xia San Li	Lateral 3 Mile Below Lateral 3 Mile	0.5-1.0 cun 0.5-1.0 cun	Perpendicular insertion. You can also Micro-puncture.
	88.17 88.18 88.19	Zi Ma Zhong Zi Ma Shang Zi Ma Xia	Center 4 Horses Upper 4 Horses Lower 4 Horses	0.8-2.5 cun 0.8-2.5 cun 0.8-2.5 cun	Perpendicular insertion
Early ejaculation	77.21	Ren Huang	Man Emperor	0.6-1.2 cun	Perpendicular insertion.
Eczema, acute	**11.17**	**Mu**	**Wood**	**0.25 cun**	**Shallow insertion, but still touch periosteum. Pinch point before insertion b/c painful.**

Notes:

25

Tung Acupuncture: A Quick Reference Guide

Indications	Point #	Name Pinyin	Name English	Insertion	Comments
Edema	**88.09** **88.10** **88.11**	**Tong Shen** **Tong Wei** **Tong Bei**	**Passing Kidney** **Passing Stomach** **Passing Back**	**0.3-0.5 cun** **0.3-0.8 cun** **0.5-1.0 cun**	**Perpendicular insertion.** **To treat edema of the face and body.** **Do not use all 6 points at the same time.**
	22.06 22.07	Zhong Bai Xia Bai	Center White Lower White	0.3-0.5 cun 0.3-0.5 cun	Perpendicular insertion.
	77.19	Di Huang	Earthly Emperor	1-1.5 cun	Perpendicular insertion. **Do not use on pregnant patient.**
	88.03	Tong Tian	Passing Sky	0.5-1.0 cun	Perpendicular insertion for leg edema
Edema of the leg	77.08 77.17 88.09 88.10 88.11	Si Hua Shang Tian Huang Tong Shen Tong Wei Tong Bei	4 Upper Flowers Heaven Emperor Passing Kidney Passing Stomach Passing Back	3.0-3.5 cun 0.5-1.0 cun 0.3-0.5 cun 0.3-0.8 cun 0.5-1.0 cun	Perpendicular insertion. To treat edema of the face and body. Do not use all 6 points (88.09-88.11) at the same time. **Do not use 77.17 on pregnant patients.**
Edema of the limbs	77.18 77.19 77.21	Shen Guan Di Huang Ren Huang	Kidney Gate Earthly Emperor Man Emperor	1.5-2.0 cun 1.0-1.5 cun 0.6-1.2 cun	Perpendicular insertion. Add 88.03 to enhance the therapeutic effect. **Do not use 77.19, 77.21 on pregnant patients.**
	88.09 88.10	Tong Shen Tong Wei	Passing Kidney Passing Stomach	0.3-0.5 cun 0.3-0.8 cun	Perpendicular insertion. Acute or chronic
Edema peripheral	**66.09**	**Shui Qu**	**Water Curve**	**0.5-1.0 cun**	**Perpendicular insertion.**
	77.11 **77.12**	**Si Hua Xia** **Fu Chang**	**4 Lower Flowers** **Bowels Intestine**	**0.5-1.0 cun** **0.5-1.0 cun**	**Perpendicular insertion.** **Use 30g-32g needle not thicker.**
Ejaculation early	L2	Shui Fu	Water Bowels	0.8-1.0 cun	Perpendicular insertion.
Elbow Golfers	**33.12** **22.08**	**Xin Men** **Wan Shun Yi**	**Heart Gate** **Wrist Flow One**	**1.0-1.5 cun** **1.0-1.5 cun**	**Perpendicular insertion. 33.12 contralateral. 22.08 Ipsilateral.**
Elbow joint pain	22.05	Ling Gu	Androit Bone	Deep insert to 22.02	Perpendicular insertion. Ipsilateral. **Do not use on pregnant patient.**
	33.07	Huo Fu Hai	Fire Bowels	0.5-1.0 cun	Perpendicular insertion. Contralateral is very effective.
	77.09	Si Huan Zhong	4 Middle Flowers	Micro-puncture	See section on micro-puncture.
	88.25	Zhong Jiu Li	Middle 9 Miles	0.8-2.0 cun	Perpendicular insertion.
Elbow pain, inner (little league pitcher's elbow)	**77.10**	**Si Hua Fu**	**4 Append Flowers**	**Micro-puncture**	**Perpendicular insertion. Add 1010.01 & 1010.08 if the condition is chronic.**
Elbow pain,(Outer) (Lateral Humeral epicondylitis)	**77.14** **77.18**	**Si Hua Wai** **Shen Guan**	**4 Lateral Flowers** **Kidney Gate**	**1.0-1.5 cun** **1.5-2.0 cun**	**Perpendicular insertion.**
Elbow tennis	DT16	Huang Ho	Paired Rivers	Micro-puncture	See section on micro-puncture.
Emphysema	**77.09** **77.10**	**Si Hua Zhong** **Si Hua Fu**	**4 Middle Flowers** **4 Append Flowers**	**Micro-puncture** **Micro-puncture**	**See section on micro-puncture.** **Right side has stronger effect.**
Emphysema	77.09 77.14	Si Hua Zhong Si Hua Wai	4 Middle Flowers 4 Lateral Flowers	Micro-puncture 1.0-1.5 cun	See section on micro-puncture. Perpendicular insertion.
Enragement, Sudden then faint	**11.15**	**Zhi Shen**	**Finger Kidney**	**0.1 cun**	**Perpenducular insertion. Use all 3 points.**

Notes:

26

Tung Acupuncture: A Quick Reference Guide

Indications	Point #	Name Pinyin	Name English	Insertion	Comments
Enteritis	11.08	Zhi Wu Jin	Finger 5 Gold	0.2-0.3 cun	Perpendicular insertion. Use both points.
	66.05	Men Jin	Door Gold	0.5 cun	Perpendicular insertion. Can also Micro-puncture. Left for males, right for females.
	77.10	Si Hua Fu	4 Append Flowers	Micro-puncture	See section on micro-puncture.
	77.11	Si Hua Xia	4 Lower Flowers	0.5-1.0 cun	Perpendicular insertion.
	77.12	Fu Chang	Bowels Intestine	0.5-1.0 cun	Use 30g-32g needle not thicker.
	L2	Shui Fu	Water Bowels	0.8-1.0 cun	Perpendicular insertion.
	VT04	Wei Mao Chi	Stomach Hair 7	Micro-puncture	See section on micro-puncture.
	VT05	Fu Chao 23	Bowel Nest 23	Micro-puncture	See section on micro-puncture.
	33.10	Chang Men	Intestine Gate	1.0-1.5 cun	Perpendicular insertion. Insertion next to the bone. **Always use left arm.**
Enteritis acute	33.10	Chang Men	Intestine Gate	1.0-1.5 cun	Perpendicular insertion. Insertion next to the bone. **Always use left arm.**
	66.05	Men Jin	Door Gold	0.5 cun	Perpendicular insertion. For male patients use left side only, for female patiens use right side. Can also Micro-puncture
	77.09	Si Hua Zhong	4 Middle Flowers	Micro-puncture	See section on micro-puncture.
	77.14	Si Hua Wai	4 Lateral Flowers	1.0-1.5 cun	Perpendicular insertion.
	77.14	Si Hua Wai	4 Lateral Flowers	1.0-1.5 cun	Perpendicular insertion. 28g needle or Micro-puncture
	77.24	Zu Qian Jin	Foot 1000 Gold	0.5-1.0 cun	Perpendicular insertion.
	77.25	Zu Wu Jin	Foot 5 Gold	0.5-1.0 cun	
	DT15	San Chiang	Three Rivers	Micro-puncture	See section on micro-puncture.
Enteritis caused by hepatitis	33.10	Chang Men	Intestine Gate	1.0-1.5 cun	Perpendicular insertion. Insertion next to the bone. **Always use left arm.**
Enteritis chronic	33.10	Chang Men	Intestine Gate	1.0-1.5 cun	Perpendicular insertion. Insert 33.10 next to the bone. **Always use left arm for 33.10.**
	77.24	Zu Qian Jin	Foot 1000 Gold	0.5-1.0 cun	
	66.05	Men Jin	Door Gold	0.5 cun	Perpendicular insertion. For male patients use left side only, for female patiens use right side. Can also Micro-puncture
Enteritis, Acute and chronic	**44.07**	**Bei Mian**	**Back Face**	**Micro-puncture**	**See section on micro-puncture.**
Enterogastritis	77.13	Si Hua Li	4 Inner Flowers	1.5-2.0 cun	Perpendicular insertion.
Enterogastritis with convulsions	77.04	Bo Qiu	Catching Ball	1.0-2.0 cun	Perpendicular insertion.
	77.09	Si Hua Zhong	4 Middle Flowers	Micro-puncture	See section on micro-puncture.
	77.14	Si Hua Wai	4 Lateral Flowers	Micro-puncture	
Entrapment neuropathy	1010.06	Hou Hui	Posterior Meetings	0.1-0.3 cun	Insertion downward. Something being pinched by soft tissue.
Epilepsy	22.08	Wan Shun Yi	Wrist Flow One	1.0-1.5 cun	Perpendicular insertion.
	22.09	Wan Shun Er	Wrist Flow Two	1.0-1.5 cun	
	55.06	Shang Liu	Upper Tumor	0.3-0.5 cun	Perpendicular insertion.
	77.18	Shen Guan	Kidney Gate	1.5-2.0 cun	

Tung Acupuncture: A Quick Reference Guide

Indications	Point #	Name Pinyin	Name English	Insertion	Comments
Epilepsy (Bilateral) (Aquired or congenital)	**88.23** **88.24**	**Jin Qian Xia** Jin Qian Shang	**Lower Gold Front** **Upper Gold Front**	**0.3-0.5 cun** **0.5-1.0 cun**	**Perpendicular insertion.**
Epilepsy, idiopathic	**77.18**	**Shen Guan**	**Kidney Gate**	**1.5-2 cun**	**Perpendicular insertion. Hereditary & trauma induced.**
Epistaxis	**22.09**	**Wan Shun Er**	Wrist Flow Two	**1.0-1.5 cun**	**Perpendicular insertion. Add 44.06**
	44.06	**Jian Zhong**	**Shoulder Center**	**1.0-1.5 cun**	**Perpendicular insertion. Add 22.09.**
	77.04	Bo Qiu	Catching Ball	1.0-2.0 cun	Perpendicular insertion. Add 22.08. Image popleteal - scapula.
Erysipelas (Skin infection)	88.01 88.02 88.03	Tong Guan Tong Shan Tong Tian	Penetrating Gate Passing Mountain Passing Sky	0.3-0.5 cun 0.5-0.8 cun 0.5-1.0 cun	Perpendicular insertion.
Erythrocytosis (Increased RBC)	**99.04**	**Tu Er**	**Earth Ear**	**0.2 cun**	Perpendicular insertion.
Erythropenia	33.11	Gan Men	Liver Gate	1.0-1.5 cun	Perpendicular insertion. Insert next to the bone. **Always use left arm.** CW= releases chest tension, CCW= for intestinal pain.
	66.06 66.07	Mu Liu Mu Dou	Wood Stay Wood Scoop	0.3-0.5 cun 0.3-0.5 cun	Perpendicular insertion.
	88.12 88.13 88.14	Ming Huang Tian Huang Qi Huang	Bright Yellow Heavenly Yellow This Yellow	1.5-2.5 cun 1.5-2.5 cun 1.5-2.0 cun	Perpendicular insertion.
Esophageal reflux	77.17	Tian Huang	Heaven Emperor	0.5-1.0 cun	Perpendicular insertion. Add 77.18. No moxa. **Do not use on pregnant patient.**
Essential tremor	**77.18**	**Shen Guan**	**Kidney Gate**	**1.5-2 cun**	**Perpendicular insertion. Add 55.06.**
Excessive stomach acid	77.17 77.18	Tian Huang Shen Guan	Heaven Emperor Kidney Gate	0.5-1.0 cun 1.5-2.0 cun	Perpendicular insertion. **Do not use 77.17 on pregnant patients.**
	88.03 88.10	Tong Tian Tong Wei	Passing Sky Passing Stomach	0.5-1.0 cun 0.3-0.8 cun	Perpendicular insertion.
Exhaustion	**1010.26**	**Ti Shen**	**Raise The Spirits**	**0.1-0.3 cun**	**Perpendicular insertion.**
Exopthalmos (Due to thyortoxicosis)	**88.17** **88.18** **88.19**	**Zi Ma Zhong** **Zi Ma Shang** **Zi Ma Xia**	**Center 4 Horses** **Upper 4 Horses** **Lower 4 Horses**	**0.8-2.5 cun.** **0.8-2.5 cun** **0.8-2.5 cun**	**Perpendicular insertion.**
Extremities pain	88.01 88.02 88.03	Tong Guan Tong Shan Tong Tian	Penetrating Gate Passing Mountain Passing Sky	0.3-0.5 cun 0.5-0.8 cun 0.5-1.0 cun	Perpendicular insertion. Only pick one or two points on one leg per treatment.
	99.03	Huo Er	Fire Ear	0.2 cun	
	1010.21 1010.22	Yu Huo Bi Yi	Jade Fire Nasal Wing	0.1-0.3 cun 0.1-0.2 cun	Perpendicular insertion. 0.5 cun lateral from nose. (Hands & feet)
Extremities weakness	1010.25	Zhou Shui	Prefect Water	0.1-0.3 cun	Insert upward or downward, use 2 needles.
Eye dark rings	**77.18**	**Shen Guan**	**Kidney Gate**	**1.5-2 cun**	**Perpendicular insertion.**
Eye diseases	Ear	Apex		Micro-puncture	See section on micro-puncture. You can also Micro-puncture the vein in back of the ear.

28

Tung Acupuncture: A Quick Reference Guide

Indications	Point #	Name Pinyin	Name English	Insertion	Comments
Eye dryness	**11.17**	**Mu**	**Wood**	**0.25 cun**	**Shallow insertion, but still touch periosteum. Pinch point before insertion b/c painful.** **Best point. Proximal point is better.**
	77.28	Guang Ming	Bright Light	0.5-1.0 cun	Perpendicular insertion. If added to other points, the treatment will be much more effective.
	88.12	Ming Huang	Bright Yellow	1.5-2.5 cun	Perpendicular insertion.
Eye jaundice	11.23	Yan Huang	Eye Yellow	0.2 cun	Perpendicular insertion.
Eye pain (Burning, tearing, eye strain)	**77.28**	**Guang Ming**	**Bright Light**	**0.5-1.0 cun**	**Perpendicular insertion.**
Eye problems	**22.08**	**Wan Shun Yi**	**Wrist Flow One**	**1.0-1.5 cun**	**Perpendicular insertion.**
Eye soreness	66.11	Hou Ju	Fire Chrysanthemum	0.5-0.8 cun	Perpendicular insertion. **Do not use on pregnant patient.**
Eye twitching	22.08 22.09	Wa Shun Yi Wan Shun Er	Wrist Flow One Wrist Flow Two	1.0-1.5 cun 1.0-1.5 cun	Perpendicular insertion.
	77.18 77.22 77.23	Shen Guan Ce San Li Ce Xia San Li	Kidney Gate Lateral 3 Mile Below Lateral 3 Mile	0.8-2.5 cun 0.5-1.0 cun 0.5-1.0 cun	Perpendicular insertion.
	88.20 88.21 88.22	Xia Quan Zhong Quan Shang Quan	Lower Fountain Middle Fountain Upper Fountain	0.3-0.5 cun 1.0-1.5 cun 1.0-1.5 cun	Perpendicular insertion.
Eye, red	**22.03**	**Shang Bai**	**Upper White**	**0.3-0.5 cun**	**Perpendicular insertion.**
Eyeball deviation	77.18 77.19 77.21	Shen Guan Di Huang Ren Huang	Kidney Gate Earthly Emperor Man Emperor	0.8-2.5 cun 1.0-1.5 cun 0.6-1.2 cun	Perpendicular insertion. **Do not use 77.19, 77.21 on pregnant patients.**
Eyelid bags	**77.18**	**Shen Guan**	**Kidney Gate**	**1.5-2 cun**	**Perpendicular insertion.**
Eyelid edema	66.11	Huo Ju	Fire Chrysanthemum	0.5-0.8 cun	Horizontal insertion. Use only one point per treatment. **Do not use on pregnant patient.**
Eyes, difficulty opening	22.14	San Cha San	Three Jam Three	1.0 – 1.5 cun	Towards the palm. Will produce immediate results.
	66.05	Men Jin	Door Gold	0.5 cun	Perpendicular insertion. For male patients use left side only, for female patiens use right side. Can also Micro-puncture
	77.21 77.28	Ren Huang Guang Ming	Man Emperor Bright Light	0.6-1.2 cun 0.5-1.0 cun	Perpendicular insertion. **Do not use 77.21 on pregnant patient.**
	88.17 88.18 88.19	Zi Ma Zhong Zi Ma Shang Zi Ma Xia	Center 4 Horses Upper 4 Horses Lower 4 Horses	0.8-2.5 cun. 0.8-2.5 cun 0.8-2.5 cun	Perpendicular insertion. (Myasthenia)

Notes:

Indications	Point #	Name Pinyin	Name English	Insertion	Comments
Facial nerve palsy	**11.14**	*Zhi San Zhong*	**Finger 3 Layer**	**0.1 cun**	**Perpenducular insertion. Use all 3 points.** **Add 77.28, 77.05 to enhance the thearaputic effect.**
	77.05 **77.06** **77.07**	**Yi Zhong** **Er Zhong** **San Zhong**	**First Weight** **Second Weight** **Third Weight**	**1.0-2.0 cun** **1.0-2.0 cun** **1.0-2.0 cun**	**Perpendicular insertion. Use all points bilaterally.** **77.05 is a projection point of 11.14.**
	77.14	Si Hua Wai	**4 Lateral Flowers**	**1.0-1.5 cun**	**Perpendicular insertion.** **28g needle or Micro-puncture**
	77.22 **77.23**	Ce San Li Ce Xia San Li	**Lateral 3 Mile** **Below Lateral 3 Mile**	0.5-1.0 cun 0.5-1.0 cun	**Perpendicular insertion.**
	88.20 **88.21**	Xia Quan Zhong Quan	**Lower Fountain** **Middle Fountain**	**0.3-0.5 cun** **1.0-1.5 cun**	**Perpendicular insertion.**
	88.22	**Shang Quan**	**Upper Fountain**	**1.0-1.5 cun**	**Perpendicular insertion.**
	88.17	Zi Ma Zhong	Center 4 Horses	0.8-2.5 cun	Perpendicular insertion.
	88.17 88.18 88.19	Zi Ma Zhong Zi Ma Shang Zi Ma Xia	Center 4 Horses Upper 4 Horses Lower 4 Horses	0.8-2.5 cun. 0.8-2.5 cun 0.8-2.5 cun	Perpendicular insertion.
	88.18	Zi Ma Shang	Upper 4 Horses	0.8-2.5 cun	Perpendicular insertion.
	88.19	Zi Ma Xia	Lower 4 Horses	0.8-2.5 cun	Perpendicular insertion.
	1010.01	Zheng Hui	Uprightness Meeting	0.1-0.3 cun	Horizontal insertion. Add 1010.08. The angle and direction of insertion is from anterior to posterior insert at an angle of 60°-90°.
	1010.17	Qi Kuai	Seven Fastness	0.5-1.5 cun	Perpendicular insertion. Treat contra lateral side.
	1010.22	Bi Yi	Nasal Wing	0.1-0.2 cun	Perpendicular insertion.
Facial numbness	77.07 77.22 77.23	San Zhong Ce San Li Ce Xia San Li	Third Weight Lateral 3 Mile Below Lateral 3 Mile	1.0-2.0 cun 0.5-1.0 cun 0.5-1.0 cun	Micro-puncture 77.07. Perpendicular insertion 77.22 & 77.23
Facial paralysis	**44.04** **44.05**	**Fu Ding** **Hou Zhi**	**Wealth Summit** **Back Branch**	**0.5 cun** **0.3-0.7 cun**	**Perpendicular insertion.**
	Ear	Apex		Micro-puncture	See section on micro-puncture.
	77.07 88.17 88.18 88.19	San Zhong Zi Ma Zhong Zi Ma Shang Zi Ma Xia	Third Weight Center 4 Horses Upper 4 Horses Lower 4 Horses	1.0-2.0 cun 0.8-2.5 cun 0.8-2.5 cun 0.8-2.5 cun	Micro-puncture 77.07, then perpendicular insertion Zi Ma points. See section on micro-puncture.
	77.14 77.22 77.23	Si Hua Wai Ce San Li Ce Xia San Li	4 Lateral Flowers Lateral 3 Mile Below Lateral 3 Mile	1.0-1.5 cun 0.5-1.0 cun 0.5-1.0 cun	Micro-puncture first, then perpendicular insertion 77.22 & 77.23. See section on micro-puncture.
	77.22	Ce San Li	Lateral 3 Mile	0.5-1.0 cun	Perpendicular (Unilateral)
	77.22 77.23	Ce San Li Ce Xia San Li	Lateral 3 Mile Below Lateral 3 Mile	0.5-1.0 cun 0.5-1.0 cun	Insert needles obliquely upwards at 45°, 2 cun, and minimum duration of 30 min. 77.22 & 77.23 contra laterally. (Chronic cases)

Tung Acupuncture: A Quick Reference Guide

Indications	Point #	Name Pinyin	Name English	Insertion	Comments
Facial spasm	22.08	Wa Shun Yi	Wrist Flow One	1.0-1.5 cun	Perpendicular insertion.
	22.09	Wan Shun Er	Wrist Flow Two	1.0-1.5 cun	
	77.22	Ce San Li	Lateral 3 Mile	0.5-1.0 cun	Perpendicular insertion.
	77.23	Ce Xia San Li	Below Lateral 3 Mile	0.5-1.0 cun	
	88.25	Zhong Jiu Li	Middle 9 Miles	0.8-2.0 cun	
	88.17	Zi Ma Zhong	Center 4 Horses	0.8-2.5 cun.	Perpendicular insertion.
	88.18	Zi Ma Shang	Upper 4 Horses	0.8-2.5 cun	
	88.19	Zi Ma Xia	Lower 4 Horses	0.8-2.5 cun	
Fainting during acupuncture	22.07	Xia Bai	Lower White	0.3-0.5 cun	Perpendicular insertion.
	22.10	Shou Jie	Hand Release	0.5 cun	
	88.28	Jie	Release Point	0.3-0.5 cun	Perpendicular insertion.
Faintness (Syncope)	1010.05	Qian Hui	Anterior Meeting	0.1-0.3 cun	Anterior to posterior. Between 1010.01 & 1010.08.
Fallopian tube blockage	11.06	Huan Chao	Return Nest	0.3 cun	Vertical insertion along bone. Either side, but not both.
Fatigue	**22.06**	**Zhong Bai**	**Center White**	**0.3-0.5 cun**	**Perpendicular insertion. Can also use 11.21, 1010.22**
	22.07	**Xia Bai**	**Lower White**	**0.3-0.5 cun**	
	44.04	**Fu Ding**	**Wealth Summit**	**0.3 cun**	**Perpendicular insertion. Can also use: 11.21, 22.06, 44.13.**
	44.13	**Zhi Tong**	**Branch Through**	**1.0 cun**	**Perpendicular insertion. Insertion along medial humerus. Add 11.21, 22.06.**
	44.14	**Luo Tong**	**Drop Through**	**0.6-1.0 cun.**	
	66.06	**Mu Liu**	**Wood Stay**	**0.3-0.5 cun**	**Perpendicular insertion.**
	66.07	**Mu Dou**	**Wood Scoop**	**0.3-0.5 cun**	
	22.14	San Cha San	Three Jam Three	1.0 – 1.5 cun	Towards the palm. Relieve fatigue
	11.21	San Yan	Three Eye	0.2 cun	Perpendicular insertion. Can also add 1010.22, 22.06. If bad tempered, add 11.17.
	22.08	Wan Shun Yi	Wrist Flow One	1.0-1.5 cun	Perpendicular insertion. (Esp. for female but only pick in one hand).
	22.09	Wan Shun Er	Wrist Flow Two	1.0-1.5 cun	
	66.10	Huo Lian	Fire Connection	0.5-0.8 cun	Horizontal insertion. Use on one side only. **Do not use on pregnant patient.**
	1010.19	Shui Tong	Water Through	0.1-0.5 cun	Horizontal insertion. Bilateral. Needle to the lateral side of chin. Add 77.18 to balance Kidney Y-Y. Bilaterally.
	1010.20	Shiu Jin	Water Gold	0.1-0.5 cun	
Feet pain	**66.04**	**Huo Zhu**	**Fire Master**	**0.3-0.8 cun**	**Perpendicular insertion. Contra lateral. Do not use on pregnant patients.**
	44.12	Li Bai	Plum White	0.5 cun	Perpendicular insertion.
Female sterility	11.24	Fu Ke	Eye Yellow	0.2 cun	Diagonal towards index finger.
Fever	DT04	Wu Ling	5 Mountain Ranges	Micro-puncture	See section on micro-puncture.
Fever of unknown origin. FUO (Infants)	**88.07**	**Gan Mao Yi**	**1st Catch Cold**	**0.8-1.5 cun**	**Perpendicular insertion.**
	88.08	**Gan Mao Er**	**2nd Catch Cold**	**0.8-1.5 cun**	

Indications	Point #	Name Pinyin	Name English	Insertion	Comments
Fever, high	**22.04**	**Da Bai**	**Big White**	Micro-puncture	**See section on micro-puncture. Perpendicular insertion. Through to 22.01 bidirectional as needed. Do not use on pregnant patients.**
	22.02	Zhong Xian	Double Saint	1.0-1.5cun	Perpendicular insertion. Needle through from 22.05 b/c palm is more painful.
Fibroids	**66.13**	**Shui Jing**	**Water Crystal**	**0.5-1.0 cun**	**Perpendicular insertion unilateral or bilateral through flexor retinaculum.**
	77.19	Di Huang	Earthly Emperor	1-1.5 cun	Perpendicular insertion. **Do not use on pregnant patient.**
Fibromylgia Due to kidney deficiency	88.09 88.10 88.11	Tong Shen Tong Wei Tong Bei	Passing Kidney Passing Stomach Passing Back	0.3-0.5 cun 0.3-0.8 cun 0.5-1.0 cun	Perpendicular insertion. Pick 2 of these 3 points (4 points at 2 thighs), Never use 3 needles same time. Pick 1 to treat the same name disease.
	1010.19 1010.20	Shui Tong Shui Jin	Water Through Water Gold	0.1-0.5 cun 0.1-0.5 cun	Horizontal insertion. Bilateral.
Finger joint pain	11.27	Wu Hu	Five Tigers	0.2 cun	Perpendicular insertion.
	33.13	Ren Shi	Human Scholar	0.5-1.0 cun	Perpendicular insertion.
Finger numbness	**66.11**	**Hou Ju**	**Fire Chrysanthemum**	**0.5-0.8 cun**	**Horizontal insertion. Do not use on pregnant patient.**
	77.18	**Shen Guan**	**Kidney Gate**	**0.8-2.5 cun**	**Perpendicular insertion. Use if there is a cervical involvement.**
	88.26 **88.27**	**Shang Jiu Li** **Xia Jiu Li**	**Upper 9 Miles** **Lower 9 Miles**	**0.8-2.0 cun** **0.8-2.0 cun**	**Perpendicular insertion.**
	11.27	Wu Hu	Five Tigers	0.2 cun	Perpendicular insertion. Contalateral.
	66.06 66.07	Mu Liu Mu Dou	Wood Stay Wood Scoop	0.3-0.5 cun 0.3-0.5 cun	Perpendicular insertion.
	DT05	Shuang Feng	Double Phoenix	Micro-puncture	See section on micro-puncture. Is done if there is a cervical involment. 7 point total.
Finger pain	**33.13**	**Ren Shi**	**Human Scholar**	**0.5-1.0 cun**	**Perpendicular insertion.**
	33.13 **66.06** **77.09**	**Ren Shi** **Mu Liu** **Si Hua Zhong**	**Human Scholar** **Wood Stay** **4 Middle Flowers**	**0.5-1.0 cun** **0.3-0.5 cun** **Micro-puncture**	**Perpendicular insertion.** **See section on micro-puncture.**
Finger pain Index finger	11.27	Wu Hu	Five Tigers	0.2 cun	Perpendicular insertion. Contra lateral.
	77.09	Si Hua Zhong	4 Middle Flowers	Micro-puncture	See section on micro-puncture.
Finger weakness	**55.03**	**Hua Gu Er**	**Flower Bone 2**	**0.5-1.0 cun**	**Perpendicular insertion. (Tremor type weakness, gripping power)**
Flatulence	**66.09**	**Shui Qu**	**Water Curve**	**0.5-1.0 cun**	**Perpendicular insertion.**
	88.26	**Shang Jiu Li**	**Upper 9 Miles**	**0.8-2.0 cun**	**Perpendicular insertion.**
	1010.10	**Si Fu Er**	**4 Bowels 2nd**	**0.1-0.2 cun**	**Horizontal insertion.**
Floating vision	88.01 88.02 88.03	Tong Guan Tong Shan Tong Tian	Penetrating Gate Passing Mountain Passing Sky	0.3-0.5 cun 0.5-0.8 cun 0.5-1.0 cun	Perpendicular insertion. Only pick one or two points on one leg per treatment.

32

Tung Acupuncture: A Quick Reference Guide

Indications	Point #	Name Pinyin	Name English	Insertion	Comments
Food poisoning	**44.07**	**Bei Mian**	**Back Face**	**0.3-0.5 cun**	**Perpendicular insertion.**
	DT01	Fen Chi Shang	Upper Separation Branch	1.0-1.5 cun	Perpendicular insertion. Bilateral. With diarrhea, add 66.05.
	DT02	Fen Chi Sha	Lower Separation Branch	0.5-1.0 cun	
Foot cramp	33.11	Gan Men	Liver Gate	1.0-1.5 cun	Perpendicular insertion. Insert next to the bone. **Always use left arm.** CW= releases chest tension, CCW= for intestinal pain.
Foot cramp	77.01	Zheng Jin	Upright Tendon	0.5-0.8 cun	Perpendicular insertion.
Foot pain	11.27	Wu Hu	Five Tigers	0.2 cun	Perpendicular insertion. 3rd & 4th point
	44.08	Ren Zong	Man Ancestor	1.2 cun	Perpendicular insertion. Caution to Biceps muscle or Cephalic vein.
	66.11	Huo Ju	Fire Chrysanthemum	0.5-0.8 cun	Horizontal insertion. Use on one side only. Metatarsal area, also foot arches issues. **Do not use on pregnant patient**
	88.25	Zhong Jiu Li	Middle 9 Miles	0.8-2.0 cun	Perpendicular insertion. Contralateral
	88.26	Shang Jiu Li	Upper 9 Miles	0.8-2.0 cun	
	88.27	Xia Jiu Li	Lower 9 Miles	0.8-2.0 cun	
Foot pain (Dorsal)	**11.27**	**Wu Hu**	**Five Tigers**	**0.2 cun**	**Perpendicular insertion. 11.27 for ligament injury. 33.08 for muscle injury.**
	33.08	**Shou Wu Jin**	**Hand Five Gold**	**0.3-0.5 cun**	**Add 44.08 & 44.12 as distal points to enhance the therapeutic effect.**
Foot soreness Difficulty walking	DT08	Jing Zhi	Essence Branch	Micro-puncture	See section on micro-puncture.
Forearm pain/cramp	33.04	Huo Chuan	Fire Threaded	0.3-0.5 cun	Perpendicular insertion.
	33.05	Huo Ling	Fire Mound	0.5-1.0 cun	Contralateral.
	33.06	Huo Shan	Fire Mountain	1.0-1.5 cun	Carple tunnel syndrome.
Fractures	**77.26**	**Qi Hu**	**Seven Tigers**	**0.5-0.8 cun**	**Perpendicular insertion.**
Frequency miscarriage.	11.06	Huan Chao	Return Nest	0.3 cun	Vertical insertion along bone. Either side, but not both.
Frequent painful urination	1010.16	Liu Kuai	Six Fastness	0.1-0.2 cun	Perpendicular insertion.
	1010.17	Qi Kuai	Seven Fastness	0.5-1.5 cun	
Frequent urination	**77.18**	**Shen Guan**	**Kidney Gate**	**0.8-2.5 cun**	**Perpendicular insertion. 77.18 first then 1010.14.**
	1010.14	**Ma Kuai Shu**	**Horse Fast Water**	**0.1-0.3 cun**	
	11.06	Huan Chao	Return Nest	0.3 cun	Vertical insertion along bone. Either side, but not both.
	66.01	Hai Bao	Seal	0.1-0.3 cun	Perpendicular insertion.
	66.02	Mu Fu	Wood Wife	0.2-0.4 cun	

Notes:

33

Tung Acupuncture: A Quick Reference Guide

Indications	Point #	Name Pinyin	Name English	Insertion	Comments
Frozen shoulder	**77.09** **77.10**	**Si Hua Zhong** **Si Hua Fu**	**4 Middle Flowers** **4 Append Flowers**	**Micro-puncture** **Micro-puncture**	**Right side has stronger effect. Add 77.13 to enhance. See section on micro-puncture.**
	77.09 **77.13** **77.14**	**Si Hua Zhong** **Si Hua Li** **Si Hua Wai**	**4 Middle Flowers** **4 Inner Flowers** **4 Lateral Flowers**	**Micro-puncture** **1.5-2.0 cun** **1.0-1.5 cun**	**Perpendicular insertion contralateral. If still can't move, micro-pucture ipsilateral.**
	44.06	Jian Zhong	Shoulder Center	1.0-1.5 cun	Perpendicular insertion.
	33.16	Qu Ling	Curved Mound	0.3-0.5 cun	Perpendicular insertion.
	55.03	Hua Gu Er	Flower Bone 2	0.5-1.0 cun	Perpendicular insertion.
	77.08 77.09	Si Hua Shang Si Hua Zhong	4 Upper Flowers 4 Middle Flowers	2.0-3.0 cun 2.0-3.0 cun	Perpendicular insertion. Either side is effective, but mostly contralateral.
	77.18	Shen Guan	Kidney Gate	0.8-2.5 cun	Perpendicular insertion. For chronic conditions add 77.25 ipsilateral. Can also Micro-punture.
	77.24 77.25	Zu Qian Jin Zu Wu Jin	Foot 1000 Gold Foot 5 Gold	0.5-1.0 cun 0.5-1.0 cun	Perpendicular insertion. Has special effect, for difficulty touhing the scapula.
	88.11	Tong Bei	Passing Back	0.5-1.0 cun	Perpendicular insertion.
Fullness in head	66.11	Huo Ju	Fire Chrysanthemum	0.5-0.8 cun	Horizontal insertion. Only one point per treatment. **Do not use on pregnant patient.**
Furunculosis	DT11	Hou Shin	Behind Heart	Micro-puncture	See section on micro-puncture. Extremities and facial area only
Galacturia	**88.09** **88.10** **88.11**	**Tong Shen** **Tong Wei** **Tong Bei**	**Passing Kidney** **Passing Stomach** **Passing Back**	**0.3-0.5 cun** **0.3-0.8 cun** **0.5-1.0 cun**	**Perpendicular insertion. Add 1010.14 to enhance the therapeutic effect.**
	77.18 77.19 77.21	Shen Guan Di Huang Ren Huang	Kidney Gate Earthly Emperor Man Emperor	0.8-2.5 cun 1.0-1.5 cun 0.6-1.2 cun	Perpendicular insertion. **Do not use 77.19, 77.21 on pregnant patients.**
	1010.14	Ma Kuai Shu	Horse Fast Water	0.1-0.3 cun	Perpendicular insertion.
Gall bladder disease	66.06	Mu Liu	Wood Stay	0.3-0.5 cun	Perpendicular insertion.
Gall stone	1010.18	Mu Zhi	Wood Branch	0.1-0.3 cun	Perpendicular insertion.
Gas poisoning (CO)	DT01 DT02	Fen Chi Shang Fen Chi Sha	Upper Separation Branch Lower Separation Branch	1.0-1.5 cun 0.5-1.0 cun	Perpendicular insertion, bilateral.
Gastric acid excessive	77.17	Tian Huang	Heaven Emperor	0.5-1 cun	Perpendicular insertion. **Do not use on pregnant patient.**
Gastric hemorrhage	88.05 88.06	Jie Mei Er Jie Mei San	Second Sister Third Sister	1.5-2.5 cun 1.5-2.5 cun	Perpendicular insertion. Always use 3 points bilaterally.
	VT04	Wei Mao Chi	Stomach Hair 7	Micro-puncture	See section on micro-puncture. Due to stress
Gastric reflux excessive	77.17	Tian Huang	Heaven Emperor	0.5-1.0 cun	Perpendicular insertion. Add 77.18 No moxa **Do not use on pregnant patient.**
Gastric ulcer	**22.11**	**Tu Shui**	**Earth Water**	**0.2-0.3 cun**	**Perpendicular insertion.**

Notes:

34

Indications	Point #	Name Pinyin	Name English	Insertion	Comments
Gastritis	**88.01** **88.02**	**Tong Guan** **Tong Shan**	**Penetrating Gate** **Passing Mountain**	**0.3-0.5 cun** **0.5-0.8 cun**	**Perpendicular insertion. Micro-puncture 77.09 first then needle 88.01 & 88.02.**
	77.08	Si Hua Shang	4 Upper Flowers	Micro-puncture	See section on micro-puncture.
	88.01 88.02 88.03	Tong Guan Tong Shan Tong Tian	Penetrating Gate Passing Mountain Passing Sky	0.3-0.5 cun 0.5-0.8 cun 0.5-1.0 cun	Perpendicular insertion.
	66.05	Men Jin	Door Gold	0.5 cun	Perpendicular insertion. Can also Micro-puncture. Left for males, right for females.
Gastritis chronic	DT11	Hou Shin	Behind Heart	Micro-puncture	See section on micro-puncture.
Gastro-enteritis	**33.16**	**Qu Ling**	**Curved Mound**	**Micro-puncture**	**See section on micro-puncture.**
Gastro-enteritis	77.04	Bo Qiu	Catching Ball	1.0-2.0 cun	Perpendicular insertion. Add 77.09. Image popleteal - scapula.
GB problems	**11.13**	**Dan**	**Gall Bladder**	**Micro-puncture**	**See section on micro-puncture.**
Giddiness (Metabolic impairment)	**33.10**	**Chang Men**	**Intestine Gate**	**1.0-1.5 cun**	**Insertion next to the bone. Intestine Gate. Always use left arm.**
Giddiness	66.03	Huo Ying	Fire Hardness	0.3-0.5 cun	Perpendicular insertion. **Do not use on pregnant patients.**
Gingivitis	**77.22** **77.23**	**Ce San Li** **Ce Xia San Li**	**Lateral 3 Mile** **Below Lateral 3 Mile**	**0.5-1.0 cun** **0.5-1.0 cun**	**Perpendicular insertion.**
Glaucoma	66.03 66.04	Hou Yin Hou Zhu	Fire Hardness Fire Master	0.3-0.5 cun 0.3-0.8 cun	Perpendicular insertion. **Do not use on pregnant patient.**
	77.18 77.19 77.21	Shen Guan Di Huang Ren Huang	Kidney Gate Earthly Emperor Man Emperor	0.8-2.5 cun 1.0-1.5 cun 0.6-1.2 cun	Perpendicular insertion. Excellent results. Added to prescription to improve therapeutic effect. **Do not use 77.19, 77.20 on a pregnant patient.**
	Ear	Apex		Micro-puncture	Also Micro-puncture back of ear. This will result in a lower intraocular pressure. See section on micro-puncture.
Glomerulonephritis (Pitting edema)	**77.17** **77.19**	**Tian Huang** **Di Huang**	**Heaven Emperor** **Earthly Emperor**	**0.5-1.0 cun** **1.0-1.5 cun**	**Perpendicular insertion.** **Do not use on pregnant patient.**
Golfers elbow	**33.12** **22.08**	**Xin Men** **Wan Shun Yi**	**Heart Gate** **Wrist Flow One**	**1.0-1.5 cun** **1.0-1.5 cun**	**Perpendicular insertion. 33.12 contralateral. 22.08 Ipsilateral.**
	77.10	**Si Hua Fu**	**4 Append Flowers**	**Micro-puncture**	**See section on micro-puncture. Add 1010.01 & 1010.08 if the condition is chronic.**
Gonorrhea	**99.02**	**Mu Er**	**Wood Ear**	**0.2 cun**	**Just touch cartilage.**
	77.19 77.21	Di Huang Ren Huang	Earthly Emperor Man Emperor	1-1.5 cun 0.6-1.2 cun	Perpendicular insertion. **Do not use on pregnant patient.**
	DT01 DT02	Fen Chi Shang Fen Chi Sha	Upper Separation Branch Lower Separation Branch	1.0-1.5 cun 0.5-1.0 cun	Perpendicular insertion. Bilateral
Gout	**11.27**	**Wu Hu**	**Five Tigers**	**0.2 cun**	**Perpendicular insertion. Needle 3rd point of Wu Hu.**

Tung Acupuncture: A Quick Reference Guide

Indications	Point #	Name Pinyin	Name English	Insertion	Comments
Governing vessel pain	**1010.27**	**Du Zong**	**Supervising Chief**	**Micro-puncture**	See section on micro-puncture.
Groin pain	**33.12** **44.10**	**Xin Men** **Tian Zong**	**Heart Gate** **Heaven Ancestor**	**1.0-1.5 cun** **1.0-1.5 cun**	**Perpendicular insertion. 33.12, close to bone only on left side. Caution to Biceps muscle or Cephalic vein.**
Gynecological problems	11.24	Fu Ke	Lady Class	0.2 cun	Diagonal towards index finger.
Haematurea	77.19	Di Huang	Earthly Emperor	1.0-1.5 cun	Perpendicular insertion. **Do not use on pregnant patient.**
Haemorrhageic disorders	55.05	Hua Gu Si	Flower Bone 4	0.5-1.0 cun	Perpendicular insertion. Use 66.08 thru to 55.05 as it hurts less.
Halitosis	DT01 DT02	Fen Chi Shang Fen Chi Sha	Upper Separation Branch Lower Separation Branch	1.0-1.5 cun 0.5-1.0 cun	Perpendicular insertion. Bilateral
Hand numbness	66.11	Huo Ju	Fire Chrysanthemum	0.5-0.8 cun	Horizontal insertion. **Use on one side only. Do not use on pregnant patient.**
	77.22 77.23	Ce San Li Ce Xia San Li	Lateral 3 Mile Below Lateral 3 Mile	0.5-1.0 cun 0.5-1.0 cun	Perpendicular insertion. Ipsilateral treatment.
Hand pain	**66.04**	**Huo Zhu**	**Fire Master**	**0.3-0.8 cun**	**Perpendicular insertion. Contra lateral. Do not use on pregnant patients.**
Hand pain (Flexor tendonitis, palm side)	**33.13** **66.04**	**Ren Shi** **Hou Zhu**	**Human Scholar** **Fire Master**	**0.5-1.0 cun** **0.3-0.8 cun**	**Perpendicular insertion. Do not use 66.04 on pregnant patient.**
Hand pain difficulty holding object	22.01 22.02	Zhong Zi Zhong Xian	Double Son Double Saint	1.0-1.5 cun 1.0-1.5 cun	Perpendicular insertion. Add 77.18 to enhance the results.
	77.18	Shen Guan	Kidney Gate	0.8-2.5 cun	Perpendicular insertion.
	77.22 77.23	Ce San Li Ce Xia San Li	Lateral 3 Mile Below Lateral 3 Mile	0.5-1.0 cun 0.5-1.0 cun	Perpendicular insertion. Contralateral.
Hand sorness	77.22 77.23	Ce San Li Ce Xia San Li	Lateral 3 Mile Below Lateral 3 Mile	0.5-1.0 cun 0.5-1.0 cun	Perpendicular insertion. Ipsilateral treatment.
Hand spasm Tendon issue	22.01 22.02	Zhong Zi Zhong Xian	Double Son Double Saint	1.0-1.5 cun 1.0-1.5 cun	Perpendicular insertion. Add 77.18 to enhance the results.
	33.16	Qu Ling	Curved Mound	0.3-0.5 cun	Perpendicular insertion. Reducing method, then needle 77.18.
Hands numbness Due to Diabetes	77.21	Ren Huang	Man Emperor	0.6-1.2 cun	Perpendicular insertion.
Hangover	**99.01**	**Er Huan**	**Ear Ring**	**0.2 cun**	**Insert from back to front of lobe towards root of the ear. Do not use with ear piercings.**
Headache Yangming & Shaoyang	77.22 77.23	Ce San Li Ce Xia San Li	Lateral 3 Mile Below Lateral 3 Mile	0.5-1.0 cun 0.5-1.0 cun	Retain 45min. Mild cases may be improvment within 2-3 Tx, Severe cases may be improvment within 4-5 Tx.
Headache Taiyang	77.18	Shen Guan	Kidney Gate	1.5-2.0 cun	Retain 45min.

36

Tung Acupuncture: A Quick Reference Guide

Indications	Point #	Name Pinyin	Name English	Insertion	Comments
Headache	**44.04** **77.18** **77.22** **77.23**	**Fu Ding** **Shen Guan** **Ce San Li** **Ce Xia San Li**	**Wealth Summit** **Kidney Gate** **Lateral 3 Mile** **Below Lateral 3 Mile**	**0.5 cun** **1.5-2.0 cun** **0.5-1.0 cun** **0.5-1.0 cun**	**Perpendicular insertion.**
	66.12	**Huo San**	**Fire Scatter**	**0.5-1.0 cun**	**Horizontal insertion. Always use with 66.10 & 66.11. Use on one side only.** **Do not use on pregnant patient.**
	77.22	**Ce San Li**	**Lateral 3 Mile**	**0.5-1.0 cun**	**Perpendicular insertion.**
	22.04 22.05	Da Bai Ling Gu	Big White Androit Bone	Deep insert to 22.01 Deep insert to 22.02	Perpendicular insertion. Adding Zhong Bai (22.06) or San Cha San 22.14 may result in a better outcome. May relieve immediately. **Do not use on pregnant patient.**
	22.04 22.14	Da Bai San Cha San	Big White Three Jam Three	Deep insert to 22.01 1.0 – 1.5 cun	Perpendicular insertion. Towards the palm. **Do not use 22.04 on pregnant patient.**
	22.08 22.09	Wan Shun Yi Wan Shun Er	Wrist Flow One Wrist Flow Two	1.0-1.5 cun 1.0-1.5 cun	Perpendicular insertion.
	33.14	Di Shi	Earth Scholar	1.0-1.5 cun	Perpendicular insertion.
	44.04 44.05	Fu Ding Hou Zhi	Wealth Summit Back Branch	0.5 cun 0.3-0.7 cun	Perpendicular insertion.
	55.06	Shang Liu	Upper Tumor	0.3-0.5 cun	Perpendicular insertion. Deep insertion may result in dyspnea & discomfort.
	66.04	Huo Zhu	Fire Master	0.3-0.8 cun	Perpendicular insertion. **Do not use on pregnant patients.**
	77.14	Si Hua Wai	4 Lateral Flowers	1.0-1.5 cun	Perpendicular insertion.
	77.23	Ce Xia San Li	Below Lateral 3 Mile	0.5-1.0 cun	Perpendicular insertion.
	88.23 88.24	Jin Qian Xia Jin Qian Shang	Lower Gold Front Upper Gold Front	0.3-0.5 cun 0.5-1.0 cun	Perpendicular insertion.
	1010.09	Shang Li	Upper Mile	0.1-0.2 cun	Embedding needle. Horizontal insertion to 1010.01 or 1010.08.
	1010.10 1010.11	Si Fu Er Si Fu Yi	4 Bowels 2nd 4 Bowels 1st	0.1-0.2 cun 0.1-0.2 cun	Horizontal insertion for 1010.10. Insertion 1010.11 towards 1010.10.
	L2	Shui Fu	Water Bowels	0.8-1.0 cun	Perpendicular insertion.
	DT04	Wu Ling	5 Mountain Ranges	Micro-puncture	See section on micro-puncture.
	DT17	Chong Xiao	Expanding Heaven	Micro-puncture	See section on micro-puncture.
Headache d/t Heart disease	66.04	Huo Zhu	Fire Master	0.3-0.8 cun	Perpendicular insertion. No moxa. **Do not use on pregnant patient.**
Headache Due to common cold	22.04	Da Bai	Big White	Deep insert to 22.01	Perpendicular insertion. **Do not use on pregnant patient.**
	DT03	Chi Shing	Seven Stars	Micro-puncture	See section on micro-puncture.
Headache tension (Frontal to temporal)	1010.05	Qian Hui	Anterior Meeting	0.1-0.3 cun	Insertion, anterior to posterior. Between 1010.01 & 1010.08.

37

© **Theodore L. Zombolas PhD (AM), LAc, Dipl.Ac. (NCCAOM).** ©

Tung Acupuncture: A Quick Reference Guide

Indications	Point #	Name Pinyin	Name English	Insertion	Comments
Headache: Migraines pain at Taiyang (Also Yangming)	**66.05**	**Men Jin**	**Door Gold**	**0.5 cun**	**Perpendicular insertion. Very effective. For male patients use left side only, for female patiens use right side. Can also Micro-puncture**
Headache: Migraines, disorders of Yangming and/or Shaoyang	77.22 77.23	Ce San Li Ce Xia San Li	Lateral 3 Mile Below Lateral 3 Mile	0.5-1.0 cun 0.5-1.0 cun	Perpendicular insertion.
Headache: Frontal	**77.17** **77.18**	**Tian Huang** **Shen Guan**	**Heaven Emperor** **Kidney Gate**	**0.5-1.0 cun** **1.5-2.0 cun**	**Perpendicular insertion. Very effective** **Do not use 77.17 on pregnant patient.**
	11.27	Wu Hu	Five Tigers	0.2 cun	Perpendicular insertion.
	55.02	Hua Gu Yi	Flower Bone 1	0.5-1.0 cun	Perpendicular insertion, 30g or 32g needle. Equivalent to 22.05. Mainly frontal, tension, HTN, migraine use 2-3 points.
	66.11	Hou Ju	Fire Chrysanthemum	0.5-0.8 cun	Horizontal insertion. May stop pain insGall BladderGall Bladdereously. **Do not use on pregnant patient.**
	77.09	Si Hua Zhong	4 Middle Flowers	Micro-puncture	See section on micro-puncture.
Headache: Migraines	66.09	Shui Qu	Water Curve	0.5-1.0 cun	Perpendicular insertion.
	77.07 77.14	San Zhong Si Hua Wai	Third Weight 4 Lateral Flowers	1.0-2.0 cun 1.0-1.5 cun	Perpendicular insertion. Micro-punture 77.07, may stop pain immediately
	88.25	**Zhong Jiu Li**	**Middle 9 Miles**	**0.8-2.0 cun**	**Perpendicular insertion.** **All types of pain of the Shaoyang channel.**
Headache: Occipital	DT17	Chong Xiao	Expanding Heaven	Micro-puncture	See section on micro-puncture.
	77.01 77.02	Zheng Jin Zheng Zong	Upright Tendon Uprightness Ancestry	0.5-0.8 cun 0.5-0.8 cun	Perpendicular insertion.
Hearing impairment	**22.05**	**Ling Gu**	**Android Bone**	**Deep insert to 22.02**	**Perpendicular insertion. Through to 22.02.** **Do not use on pregnant patient.**
Hearing loss	**88.17** **88.18** **88.19**	**Zi Ma Zhong** **Zi Ma Shang** **Zi Ma Xia**	**Center 4 Horses** **Upper 4 Horses** **Lower 4 Horses**	**0.8-2.5 cun.** **0.8-2.5 cun** **0.8-2.5 cun**	**Perpendicular insertion.**
Heart beat (Abnormal)	11.19	Xin Chang	Heart Normal	0.1-0.2 cun	Perpendicular insertion, use both points.
Heart disease	**88.01** **88.02** **88.03**	**Tong Guan** **Tong Shan** **Tong Tian**	**Penetrating Gate** **Passing Mountain** **Passing Sky**	**0.3-0.5 cun** **0.5-0.8 cun** **0.5-1.0 cun**	**Perpendicular insertion.** **Only pick one or two points on one leg per treatment.**
	77.09 77.14	Si Hua Zhong Si Hua Wai	4 Middle Flowers 4 Lateral Flowers	Micro-puncture 1.0-1.5 cun	Micro-punctureting is effective. See section on micro-puncture.
Heart failure	11.15	Zhi Shen	Finger Kidney	0.1 cun	Perpenducular insertion. Use all 3 points.
Heart palpitations	**33.16**	**Qu Ling**	**Curved Mound**	**Micro-puncture**	**See section on micro-puncture.**
Heart paralysis (For resuscitation)	**66.03** **66.04**	**Huo Ying** **Huo Zhu**	**Fire Hardness** **Fire Master**	**0.3-0.5 cun** **0.3-0.8 cun**	**Perpendicular insertion.** **Do not use on pregnant patients.**

Tung Acupuncture: A Quick Reference Guide

Indications	Point #	Name Pinyin	Name English	Insertion	Comments
Heart weakness Due to Hypertension.	66.10	Huo Lian	Fire Connection	0.5-0.8 cun	Horizontal insertion. **Do not use on pregnant patients.**
Heavy para-spinal pain (low back and back).	22.08 22.09	Wan Shun Yi Wan Shun Er	Wrist Flow One Wrist Flow Two	1.0-1.5 cun 1.0-1.5 cun	Perpendicular insertion. (Esp. for female but only pick in one hand).
Heel pain	**11.27**	**Wu Hu**	**Five Tigers**	**0.2 cun**	**Perpendicular insertion. Needle all 5 points**
	11.27 **88.16**	**Wu Hu** **Huo Quan**	**Five Tigers** **Fire Complete**	**0.2 cun** **1.5-2.0 cun**	**Perpendicular insertion.** **88.16 is a sGall Bladderdby point.**
	22.05	**Lin Gu**	**Androit Bone**	**Deep insert to 22.02**	**Perpendicular insertion. Needle along the bone. Do not use on pregnant patient.**
	77.09 77.11	Si Hua Zhong Si Hua Xia	4 Middle Flowers 4 Lower Flowers	Micro-puncture 0.5-1.0 cun	Perpendicular insertion along the bone. Use thin needles with 77.11. See section on micro-puncture.
	88.14 88.15 88.16	Qi Huang Huo Zhi Huo Quan	This Yellow Fire Branch Fire Complete	1.5-2.0 cun 1.5-2.0 cun 1.5-2.0 cun	Perpendicular insertion.
	88.15 88.16	Huo Zhi Huo Quan	Fire Branch Fire Complete	1.5-2.0 cun 1.5-2.0 cun	Perpendicular insertion.
	88.16	Huo Quan	Fire Complete	1.5-2.0 cun	Perpendicular insertion.
	1010.06	Hou Hui	Posterior Meetings	0.1-0.3 cun	Insert downward.
Heel spurs	77.09 77.11	Si Hua Zhong Si Hua Xia	4 Middle Flowers 4 Lower Flowers	Micro-puncture 0.5-1.0 cun	See section on micro-puncture. Perpendicular insertion. Insert needle close to the Tibia. "Like treats like". Use thin needles with 77.11. Add 33.12 to improve the therapeutic effect.
Hematuria	77.18 77.19 77.21	Shen Guan Di Huang Ren Huang	Kidney Gate Earthly Emperor Man Emperor	0.8-2.5 cun 1.0-1.5 cun 0.6-1.2 cun	Perpendicular insertion. **Do not use 77.19, 77.21 on pregnant patients.**
Hemianesthesia	DT04	Wu Ling	5 Mountain Ranges	Micro-puncture	See section on micro-puncture.

Notes:

39

Indications	Point #	Name Pinyin	Name English	Insertion	Comments
Hemiplegia	11.10	Mu Huo	Wood Fire	0.1 cun	Insert from Ulnar to Radial side. 3 Tx. 5 days apart. Do not exceed 5 min for 1st TX, 3 min for 2nd TX and 1 min for 3rd Tx. Use 11.10 first then add 22.04, 22.05
	22.04 22.05	Da Bai Ling Gu	Big White Androit Bone	Deep insert to 22.01 Deep insert to 22.02	Perpendicular insertion. Add 11.10 to enhance the thereaputic effect. Do not use on pregnant patient.
	44.06	Jian Zhong	Shoulder Center	1.0-1.5 cun	Perpendicular insertion. Contra lateral.
	88.25	Zhong Jiu Li	Middle 9 Miles	0.8-2.0 cun	Perpendicular insertion. Right side is more powerful than left side. Treat bilateral. (Left hemiplegia is more difficult to treat)
	88.25 88.26 88.27	Zhong Jiu Li Shang Jiu Li Xia Jiu Li	Middle 9 Miles Upper 9 Miles Lower 9 Miles	0.8-2.0 cun 0.8-2.0 cun 0.8-2.0 cun	Perpendicular insertion. Add 1010.01 and 1010.06
	1010.22	Bi Yi	Nasal Wing	0.1-0.2 cun	Perpendicular insertion.
	22.01 22.02	Zhong Zi Zhong Xian	Double Son Double Saint	1.0-1.5 cun 1.0-1.5 cun	Perpendicular insertion.
	22.05	Ling Gu	Androit Bone	Deep insert to 22.02	Perpendicular insertion. Bidirectional as needed. Do not use on pregnant patient.
	44.15	Xia Qu	Lower Curve	0.6-1.0 cun	Perpendicular insertion.
	77.18	Shen Guan	Kidney Gate	0.8-2.5 cun	Perpendicular insertion.
	88.17 88.18 88.19	Zi Ma Zhong Zi Ma Shang Zi Ma Xia	Center 4 Horses Upper 4 Horses Lower 4 Horses	0.8-2.5 cun. 0.8-2.5 cun 0.8-2.5 cun	Perpendicular insertion.
	88.29 88.30 88.31	Nei Tong Guan Nei Tong Shan Nei Tong Tian	Inner Passing Gate Inner Passing Mountain Inner Passing Sky	1.0 cun 1.0 cun 1.0 cun	Perpendicular insertion.
	1010.01	Zheng Hui	Uprightness Meeting	0.1-0.3 cun	Horizontal insertion. Add 1010.08. Angle and direction of insertion is anterior to posterior insert 60°-90°.
	1010.02 1010.03 1010.04	Zhou Yuan Zhou Kun Zhou Lun	Prefecture Round Prefecture Elder Brother Prefecture Mountain	0.1-0.3 cun 0.1-0.3 cun 0.1-0.3 cun	Horizontal insertion.
	1010.06	Hou Hui	Posterior Meetings	0.1-0.3 cun	Insertion downward.
	DT04	Wu Ling	5 Mountain Ranges	Micro-puncture	See section on micro-puncture.
	DT11	Hou Shin	Behind Heart	Micro-puncture	See section on micro-puncture.
Hemiplegia due to K deficiency	77.18	Shen Guan	Kidney Gate	0.8-2.5 cun	Perpendicular insertion.
	1010.19 1010.20	Shui Tong Shiu Jin	Water Through Water Gold	0.1-0.5 cun 0.1-0.5 cun	Horizontal insertion. Bilateral.
Hemorrhagic disorders	66.08	Liu Wan	Sixth Finish	0.3-0.5 cun	Perpendicular insertion. Do not use with lung disease

Tung Acupuncture: A Quick Reference Guide

Indications	Point #	Name Pinyin	Name English	Insertion	Comments
Hemorrhoid pain (Internal external)	33.01 33.02 33.03	Qi Men Qi Jiao Qi Zheng	This Door This Corner This Uprightness	0.2-0.5 cun 0.2-0.5 cun 0.2-0.5 cun	Horizontal insertion. Use 3 needles total, 33.01-33.03. Insert in one side L or R. Can also Micro-puncture (Micro-puncture Popleteal area first, then needle these 3 points.)
Hepatalgia (Liver pain)	**99.02**	**Mu Er**	**Wood Ear**	**0.2 cun**	**Just touch cartilage.**
Hepatitis	**11.23**	**Yan Huang**	**Eye Yellow**	**0.2 cun**	**Perpendicular insertion. Type A & B hepatitis.**
	33.11 **88.12**	**Gan Men** **Ming Huang**	**Liver Gate** **Bright Yellow**	**1.0-1.5 cun** **1.5-2.5 cun**	**Perpendicular insertion. Insert next to the bone. Always use left arm. Good for acute and chronic Hepatitis. Add 33.10 to enhance the therapeutic effect.**
	88.12 88.13 88.14	Ming Huang Tian Huang Qi Huang	Bright Yellow Heavenly Yellow This Yellow	1.5-2.5 cun 1.5-2.5 cun 1.5-2.0 cun	Perpendicular insertion.
Hepatitis A	**88.12** **88.13** **88.14**	**Ming Huang** **Tian Huang** **Qi Huang**	**Bright Yellow** **Heavenly Yellow** **This Yellow**	**1.5-2.5 cun** **1.5-2.5 cun** **1.5-2.0 cun**	**Perpendicular insertion. Insertion bi lateral.**
	88.15 **88.16**	**Huo Zhi** **Huo Quan**	**Fire Branch** **Fire Complete**	**1.5-2.0 cun** **1.5-2.0 cun**	**Perpendicular insertion.**
	11.20	Mu Yan	Wood Inflammation	0.2 cun	Perpendicular insertion. If bad tempered, add 11.17.
Hepatitis acute	**33.11**	**Gan Men**	**Liver Gate**	**1.0-1.5 cun**	**Perpendicular insertion. Insert next to the bone. Always use left arm. CW= releases chest tension, CCW= for intestinal pain.**
	33.10 33.11	Chang Men Gan Men	Intestine Gate Liver Gate	1.0-1.5 cun 1.0-1.5 cun	Perpendicular insertion. Insert next to the bone. **Always use left arm.**
Hepatitis chronic with jaundice	88.12 88.13 88.14	Ming Huang Tian Huang Qi Huang	Bright Yellow Heavenly Yellow This Yellow	1.5-2.5 cun 1.5-2.5 cun 1.5-2.0 cun	Perpendicular insertion.
Hepatomegaly	**99.02**	**Mu Er**	**Wood Ear**	**0.2 cun**	**Just touch cartilage.**
	11.20	Mu Yan	Wood Inflammation	0.2 cun	Perpendicular insertion. If bad tempered, add 11.17
Hernia	11.01 11.02 11.03 11.04 11.05	Da Jian Xiao Jian Fu Jian Wai Jian Zhong Jian	Big Distance Small Distance Floating Distance External Distance Center Distance	0.2-0.3 cun 0.2-0.3 cun 0.1-0.2 cun 0.1-0.2 cun 0.2-0.3 cun	All points perpenducular. Needle 2-3 points from this group of points. This is good for a hernia up to the size of a dime. Apply to right side. Best combination is 11.01, 11.02 & 11.05.
	1010.15	Fu Kuai	Bowels Ease	0.1-0.3 cun	Perpendicular insertion.
Hernia of the large intestine	11.17	Mu	Wood	0.25 cun	Shallow insertion, but still touch periosteum. Pinch point before insertion b/c painful.
Hernia pain	**11.03** **11.04** **66.01**	**Fu Jian** **Wai Jian** **Hai Bao**	**Floating Distance** **External Distance** **Seal**	**0.1-0.2 cun** **0.1-0.2 cun** **0.1-0.3 cun**	**Perpendicular insertion.**
Herpes zoster	11.26	Zhi Wu	Control Dirt	Micro-puncture	See section on micro-puncture.

41

Indications	Point #	Name Pinyin	Name English	Insertion	Comments
Hiccup	1010.19 1010.20	Shui Tong Shiu Jin	Water Through Water Gold	0.1-0.5 cun 0.1-0.5 cun	Horizontal insertion. Bilaterally. Needle to the lateral side of chin. Add 77.18 to balance Kidney Y-Y. Most effective for intractable hiccup.
Hidrosis	Ear	Apex		Micro-puncture	Is very effective.
High fever	**22.02**	**Zhong Xian**	**Double Saint**	**1.0-1.5 cun**	**Perpendicular insertion.**
	22.04	Da Bai	Big White	Micro-puncture	See section on micro-puncture. **Do not use on pregnant patients.**
	99.04	Tu Er	Earth Ear	0.2 cun	Perpendicular insertion.
High fever in children	DT03	Chi Shing	Seven Stars	Micro-puncture	See section on micro-puncture.
Hip pain	**22.09**	**Wan Shun Er**	**Wrist Flow Two**	**1.0-1.5 cun**	**Perpendicular insertion.**
	33.12 **77.20**	**Xin Men** **Si Zhi**	**Heart Gate** **Four Limbs**	**1.0-1.5 cun** **1-1.5 cun**	**Perpendicular insertion.** **Do not use 77.20 pregnant patient.**
Hoarseness (Loss of voice)	**44.07**	**Bei Mian**	**Back Face**	**0.3-0.5 cun**	**Perpendicular insertion.**
	88.32	**Shi Yin**	**Shih-Yin**	**1.0-1.5 cun**	**Horizontal insertion. Bilateral. Keep knee at 90° angle and have patient swallow for induction.**
Hydrocephalus	**55.06**	**Shang Liu**	**Upper Tumor**	**0.3-0.5 cun**	**Perpendicular insertion. Do not make deep insertion = dyspnea & discomfort.**
	77.01	**Zheng Jin**	**Upright Tendon**	**0.5-0.8 cun**	**Perpendicular insertion. Through the Achilles tendon. Add 55.06. Contra lateral insertion first, then ipsi lateral insertion. Always use 77.01 with 77.02 for better results.**
	77.01 55.06	Zheng Jin Shang Liu	Upright Tendon Upper Tumor	0.5-0.8 cun 0.3-0.5 cun	Perpendicular insertion. May have a favorable effect. Micro-punctureting at 77.07 San Zhong may produce a better result.
	77.01 77.02	Zheng Jin Zheng Zong	Upright Tendon Uprightness Ancestry	0.5-0.8 cun 0.5-0.8 cun	Perpendicular insertion. (Penetrate tendon more effective). Needle robust patient in a sitting position; weak person with side lying position.
Hyper thyroidism	**77.05** **77.06** **77.07**	**Yi Zhong** **Er Zhong** **San Zhong**	**First Weight** **Second Weight** **Third Weight**	**1.0-2.0 cun** **1.0-2.0 cun** **1.0-2.0 cun**	**Perpendicular insertion. Clinically tend to use the right side. 77.05 projection point of 11.14.**
Hyperactivity of liver-fire and irritability	11.17	Mu	Wood	0.25 cun	Shallow insertion, but still touch periosteum. Pinch point before insertion b/c painful.
Hyperchlorhydria (Excessive gastric acid)	77.17 77.18	Tian Huang Shen Guan	Heaven Emperor Kidney Gate	1.5-2 cun 0.5-1 cun	Perpendicular insertion. **Do not use 77.17 on pregnant patient.**
	77.17	Tian Huang	Heaven Emperor	0.5-1.0	Perpendicular insertion. No moxa. **Do not use on pregnant patient.**
Hyperemia (High fever)	99.04	Tu Er	Earth Ear	0.2 cun	Perpendicular insertion.
Hyperhydrosis	**11.17**	**Mu**	**Wood**	**0.25 cun**	**Shallow insertion, but still touch periosteum. Pinch point before insertion b/c painful.**

42

Tung Acupuncture: A Quick Reference Guide

Indications	Point #	Name Pinyin	Name English	Insertion	Comments
Hyper-Leucocytosis	**88.12** **88.13** **88.14**	**Ming Huang** **Tian Huang** **Qi Huang**	**Bright Yellow** **Heavenly Yellow** **This Yellow**	**1.5-2.5 cun** **1.5-2.5 cun** **1.5-2.0 cun**	**Perpendicular insertion.**
	66.06 66.07	Mu Liu Mu Dou	Wood Stay Wood Scoop	0.3-0.5 cun 0.3-0.5 cun	Perpendicular insertion.
	77.18 77.19 77.21	Shen Guan Di Huang Ren Huang	Kidney Gate Earthly Emperor Man Emperor	0.8-2.5 cun 1.0-1.5 cun 0.6-1.2 cun	Perpendicular insertion. Tonify both the Kidney & Spleen. **Do not use 77.19, 77.21 on pregnant patients.**
Hypertension	22.06 22.07	Zhong Bai Xia Bai	Center White Lower White	Micro-puncture 0.3-0.5 cun	See section on micro-puncture. Perpendicular insertion for 22.07.
	44.02 **44.03**	**Hou Zhui** **Shou Ying**	**Back Vertibrae** **Head Wisdom**	**0.3-0.5 cun** **0.3-0.5 cun**	**Perpendicular insertion.**
	44.04 **44.05**	**Fu Ding** **Hou Zhi**	**Wealth Summit** **Back Branch**	**0.5 cun** **0.3-0.7 cun**	**Perpendicular insertion.** **Can also add: 44.13, 44.14.**
	44.13 **44.14** **44.15**	**Zhi Tong** **Luo Tong** **Xia Qu**	**Branch Through** **Drop Through** **Lower Curve**	**1 cun** **0.6-1.0 cun** **0.6-1.0 cun**	**Perpendicular insertion.** **Insertion along medial humerus.**
	44.16	**Shang Qu**	**Upper Curve**	**0.6-1.5 cun**	**Perpendicular insertion.**
	77.14	**Si Hua Wai**	**4 Lateral Flowers**	**1.0-1.5 cun**	**Perpendicular insertion, use 28g needle or Micro-puncture**
	77.17	**Tian Huang**	**Heaven Emperor**	**0.5-1.0 cun**	**Perpendicular insertion.** **Do not use on pregnant patient.**
	66.03 66.11	Huo Ying Huo Ju	Fire Hardness Fire Chrysanthemum	0.3-0.5 cun 0.5-0.8 cun	Perpendicular insertion. **Do not use 66.11 on pregnant patient.**
	66.11	Huo Ju	Fire Chrysanthemum	0.5-0.8 cun	Horizontal insertion. **Use on one side only.** **Do not use on pregnant patient.**
	77.09 77.14	Si Hua Zhong Si Hua Wai	4 Middle Flowers 4 Lateral Flowers	Micro-puncture 0.5-1.0 cun	See section on micro-puncture. Perpendicular insertion.
	88.01 88.02 88.03	Tong Guan Tong Shan Tong Tian	Penetrating Gate Passing Mountain Passing Sky	0.3-0.5 cun. 0.3-0.5 cun 0.5-1.0 cun	Perpendicular insertion. Only bleed one point in each thigh to treat hypertension. Only pick one or two points on one leg per treatment.
	DT04	Wu Ling	5 Mountain Ranges	Micro-puncture	See section on micro-puncture.
	Ear	Tip		Micro-puncture	See section on micro-puncture.
Hypertension renal	77.18	Shen Guan	Kidney Gate	0.8-2.5 cun	Perpendicular insertion.
Hypochondriac pain	22.14	San Cha San	Three Jam Three	1.0 – 1.5 cun	Towards the palm.
Hypodermic injection pain	**88.28**	**Jie**	**Release Point**	**0.3-0.5 cun**	**Perpendicular insertion.**
Hysteria	**11.13**	**Dan**	**Gall Bladder**	**Micro-puncture**	**See section on micro-puncture.**
	77.18	**Shen Guan**	**Shen-Kuan**	**0.8-2.5 cun**	**Perpendicular insertion.**
	1010.08	**Zhen Jing**	**Tranquility**	**0.1-0.2 cun**	**Insert towards nose. Always use with 1010.01.**
	99.04	Tu Er	Earth Ear	0.2 cun	
	1010.18	Mu Zhi	Wood Branch	0.1-0.3 cun	Perpendicular insertion.

43

Tung Acupuncture: A Quick Reference Guide

Indications	Point #	Name Pinyin	Name English	Insertion	Comments
Hysteromyoma	11.06	Huan Chao	Return Nest	0.3 cun	All points perpenducular.
	88.04	Jie Mei Yi	First Sister	1.5-2.0 cun	Either side for 11.06, but not both.
	88.05	Jie Mei Er	Second Sister	1.5-2.5 cun	All other points bilaterally.
	88.06	Jie Mei San	Third Sister	1.5-2.5 cun	
	11.24	Fu Ke	Lady Class	0.2 cun	Diagonal towards index finger. Add 11.06 to enhance the therapeutic effect.
	22.01	Zhong Zi	Double Son	1.0-1.5 cun	Perpendicular insertion.
	22.02	Zhong Xian	Double Saint	1.0-1.5 cun	
Impact injury	**22.03**	**Shang Bai**	**Upper White**	**0.3-0.5 cun**	**Perpendicular insertion.**
Impact trauma	**77.26**	**Qi Hu**	**Seven Tigers**	**0.5-0.8 cun**	**Perpendicular insertion. Use all 3 points at same time contra lateral. Similar to 5 tigers 11.27.**
Impotence	77.19	Di Huang	Earthly Emperor	1.0-1.5 cun	Perpendicular insertion.
	77.21	Ren Huang	Man Emperor	0.6-1.2 cun	Perpendicular insertion.
	88.09	Tong Shen	Passing Kidney	0.3-0.5 cun	Perpendicular insertion. Pick 2 of these 3 points (4 points at 2 thighs), Never use 3 needles same time.
	88.10	Tong Wei	Passing Stomach	0.3-0.8 cun	
	88.11	Tong Bei	Passing Back	0.5-1.0 cun	
	L2	Shui Fu	Water Bowels	0.8-1.0 cun	Perpendicular insertion.
Impotence & Premature ejaculation	**77.19**	**Di Huang**	**Earthly Emperor**	**1.0-1.5 cun**	**Perpendicular insertion.**
Index finger pain	66.01	Hai Bao	Seal	0.1-0.3 cun	Perpendicular insertion, contra lateral.
Indigestion	**66.07**	**Mu Dou**	**Wood Scoop**	**0.3-0.5 cun**	**Perpendicular insertion.**
	66.09	**Shui Qu**	**Water Curve**	**0.5-1.0 cun**	**Perpendicular insertion.**
	88.12	**Ming Huang**	**Bright Yellow**	**1.5-2.5 cun**	**Perpendicular insertion.**
	88.13	**Tian Huang**	**Heavenly Yellow**	**1.5-2.5 cun**	**Insertion bi lateral.**
	88.14	**Qi Huang**	**This Yellow**	**1.5-2.0 cun**	
	66.06	Mu Liu	Wood Stay	0.3-0.5 cun	Perpendicular insertion.
	VT03	King Wu	Gold Five	Micro-puncture	See section on micro-puncture.
Infections parotitis (mumps)	**77.27**	**Wai San Guan**	**Outer 3 Gates**	**1.0-1.5 cun.**	**Perpendicular insertion. Similar to 5 tigers 11.27.**
Infertility	**11.06**	**Huan Chao**	**Return Nest**	**0.3 cun**	**Vertical insertion along bone. Either side, but not both.**
	66.02	**Mu Fu**	**Wood Wife**	**0.2-0.4 cun**	**Perpendicular insertion. Use 30g-32g needle. Touch periosteum. For female infertility, add 77.17, 77.18. If stressed add 1010.01, 1010.08.**
	11.24	Fu Ke	Lady Class	0.2 cun	Diagonal towards index finger.
	11.06	Huan Chao	Return Nest	0.3 cun	11.24 Diagonal towards index finger. Bilaterally for effective results. Treat daily or every other day. 11.06 use either side, but not both. Chronic.
	11.24	Fu Ke	Lady Class	0.2 cun	
Inflammation	**11.06**	**Huan Chao**	**Return Nest**	**0.3 cun**	**Vertical insertion along bone. Either side, but not both.**
Influenza	**22.01**	**Zhong Zi**	**Double Son**	**1.0-1.5cun**	**Perpendicular insertion.**
	88.07	**Gan Mao Yi**	**1st Catch Cold**	**0.8-1.5 cun**	**Perpendicular insertion. Can add 1010.22.**
	88.08	**Gan Mao Er**	**2nd Catch Cold**	**0.8-1.5 cun**	

44

© **Theodore L. Zombolas PhD** (AM), **LAc, Dipl.Ac.** (NCCAOM). ©

Tung Acupuncture: A Quick Reference Guide

Indications	Point #	Name Pinyin	Name English	Insertion	Comments
Inguinal hernia	**11.01** **11.02** **11.03** **11.04**	**Da Jian** **Xiao Jian** **Fu Jian** **Wai Jian**	**Big Distance** **Small Distance** **Floating Distance** **External Distance**	**0.2-0.3 cun** **0.2-0.3 cun** **0.1-0.2 cun** **0.1-0.2 cun**	**All points perpenducular. Apply to right side. Dime size hernia can be reduced with acupuncture, 2-3 weeks 1Tx/wk. Greater size requires surgery. Best combination is 11.01 & 11.02. Use 2-3 points.**
	66.01	Hai Bao	Seal	0.1-0.3 cun	Perpendicular insertion, contra lateral.
Inguinal pain (Due to ishemia)	**33.12**	**Xin Men**	**Heart Gate**	**1.0-1.5 cun**	**Perpendicular insertion. Insert next to the bone. Always use left arm.**
Insomnia	**22.04** **88.25** **88.26** **88.27**	**Da Bai** **Zhong Jiu Li** **Shang Jiu Li** **Xia Jiu Li**	**Big White** **Middle 9 Miles** **Upper 9 Miles** **Lower 9 Miles**	Deep insert to 22.01 **0.8-2.0 cun** **0.8-2.0 cun** **0.8-2.0 cun**	**Perpendicular insertion. Do not use 22.04 on pregnant patients.**
	77.17	**Tian Huang**	**Heaven Emperor**	**0.5-1.0 cun**	**Perpendicular insertion. Do not use on pregnant patient.**
	1010.08	**Zhen Jing**	**Tranquility**	**0.1-0.2 cun**	**Insert towards nose. Always use with 1010.01.**
	Ear	Apex		Micro-puncture	See section on micro-puncture.
	77.18 77.19 77.21 1010.08	Shen Guan Di Huang Ren Huang Zhen Jing	Kidney Gate Earthly Emperor Man Emperor Tranquility	0.8-2.5 cun 1.0-1.5 cun 0.6-1.2 cun 0.1-0.2 cun	Perpendicular insertion. **Do not use 77.19, 77.21 on pregnant patients.**
	L2	Shui Fu	Water Bowels	0.8-1.0 cun	Perpendicular insertion.
Intentional tremor	**77.18**	**Shen Guan**	**Kidney Gate**	**0.8-2.5 cun**	**Perpendicular insertion. Add 55.06.**
	55.06	Shang Liu	Upper Tumor	0.3-0.5 cun	Perpendicular insertion. Deep insertion may result in dyspnea & discomfort.
Intercostal neuralgia (Shingles etc..)	**77.14**	**Si Hua Wai**	**4 Lateral Flowers**	**1.0-1.5 cun**	**Perpendicular insertion 28g or you can Micro-puncture Add 22.05. Micro-punture black blood to treat acute enteritis, intercostals neuralgia, chest oppression, asthma, sciatica (along GB meridian) and other neuralgia.**
	88.17 88.18 88.19	Zi Ma Zhong Zi Ma Shang Zi Ma Xia	Center 4 Horses Upper 4 Horses Lower 4 Horses	0.8-2.5 cun. 0.8-2.5 cun 0.8-2.5 cun	Perpendicular insertion. This is also good for pain in the chest costal area and abdomen. If the syptoms are bilateral, use up to 6 needles.
Internal organ disease	77.09 77.14	Si Hua Zhong Si Hua Wai	4 Middle Flowers 4 Lateral Flowers	Micro-puncture 0.5-1.0 cun	See section on micro-puncture. Perpendicular insertion.
Intestine Pain.	33.11	Gan Men	Liver Gate	1.0-1.5 cun	Perpendicular insertion. Insert next to the bone. **Always use left arm.** CW= releases chest tension, CCW= for intestinal pain.
Intraductal papillomas	77.05 77.06 77.07	Yi Zhong Er Zhong San Zhong	First Weight Second Weight Third Weight	1.0-2.0 cun 1.0-2.0 cun 1.0-2.0 cun	Perpendicular insertion. Use all points bilaterally. 77.05 projection point of 11.14.

45

Tung Acupuncture: A Quick Reference Guide

Indications	Point #	Name Pinyin	Name English	Insertion	Comments
Irregular menstruation	**11.24**	**Fu Ke**	**Lady Class**	**0.2 cun**	**Diagonal towards index finger.**
	11.06	Huan Chao	Return Nest	0.3 cun	Vertical insertion along bone. Either side, but not both.
Irritable colon	11.08	Zhi Wu Jin	Finger 5 Gold	0.2-0.3 cun	Perpendicular insertion. Use both points.
Irritable Heart Syndrome	11.02	Xiao Jian	Small Distance	0.2-0.3 cun	Perpendicular insertion. Apply to right side.
Itching of skin due to allergies	22.14	San Cha San	Three Jam Three	1.0 – 1.5 cun	Towards the palm.
Itching skin	**11.17**	**Mu**	**Wood**	**0.25 cun**	**Shallow insertion, but still touch periosteum. Pinch point before insertion b/c painful.**
Jaundice	**33.11**	**Gan Men**	**Liver Gate**	**1.0-1.5 cun**	**Perpendicular insertion. Insert next to the bone. Always use left arm. CW= releases chest tension, CCW= for intestinal pain.**
	44.08	Ren Zong	Man Ancestor	1.2 cun	Perpendicular insertion. Caution Biceps muscle or Cephalic vein.
	88.12 88.13 88.14	Ming Huang Tian Huang Qi Huang	Bright Yellow Heavenly Yellow This Yellow	1.5-2.5 cun 1.5-2.5 cun 1.5-2.0 cun	Perpendicular insertion.
Jaundice Which induces dizziness	88.15 88.16	Huo Zhi Huo Quan	Fire Branch Fire Complete	1.5-2.0 cun 1.5-2.0 cun	Perpendicular insertion.
Jaundice due to acute Hepatitis	33.11	Gan Men	Liver Gate	1.0-1.5 cun	Perpendicular insertion. Insert next to the bone. **Always use left arm.** CW= releases chest tension, CCW= for intestinal pain.
Joint pain	22.05 66.04	Ling Gu Huo Zhu	Android Bone Fire Master	Deep insert to 22.02 0.3-0.8 cun	Perpendicular insertion. Insert needle along the bones. **Do not use these points on pregnant patient.**
	11.27	Wu Hu	Five Tigers	0.2 cun	Perpendicular insertion. Use up to 3 needles.
Joint pain Knee	33.12	Xin Men	Heart Gate	1.0-1.5 cun	On healthy side. Then needle a distal point on the diseased side as the attracting point.
Joint pain Shoulder	77.18	Shen Guan	Kidney Gate	0.8-2.5 cun	Very effective. Add the corresponding shu-stream point for better results.
Joint sublixation	**77.26**	**Qi Hu**	**Seven Tigers**	**0.5-0.8 cun**	**Perpendicular insertion. Add 44.15. Use all 3 points at same time contra lateral. Similar to 5 tigers 11.27.**
Joint swelling	11.27	Wu Hu	Five Tigers	0.2 cun	Perpendicular insertion.
Keratitis	Ear	Apex		Micro-puncture	See section on micro-puncture.
Kidney Deficiency	66.12	Huo San	Fire Scatter	0.5-1.0 cun	Horizontal insertion. **Do not use on pregnant patient.**
	77.18	Shen Guan	Kidney Gate	0.8-2.5 cun	Perpendicular insertion.
	22.08 22.09	Wan Shun Yi Wan Shun Er	Wrist Flow One Wrist Flow Two	1.0-1.5 cun 1.0-1.5 cun	Perpendicular insertion. (Esp. for female but only pick in one hand).

Tung Acupuncture: A Quick Reference Guide

Indications	Point #	Name Pinyin	Name English	Insertion	Comments
Kidney diseases	22.07	Xia Bai	Lower White	0.3-0.5 cun	Perpendicular insertion. Needle along the bone for better results.
	88.09	Tong Shen	Passing Kidney	0.3-0.5 cun	Perpendicular insertion.
	88.10	Tong Wei	Passing Stomach	0.3-0.8 cun	
	88.11	Tong Bei	Passing Back	0.5-1.0 cun	
	L1	Shui Chung	Water Center	0.8-1.0 cun	Perpendicular insertion.
	L2	Shui Fu	Water Bowels	0.8-1.0 cun	
Kidney stones	**1010.13**	**Ma Jin Shui**	**Horse Gold Water**	**0.1-0.3 cun**	**Perpendicular insertion. Right side is more effective than left side. Use right side if patient is right handed.**
Kidney symptoms	**11.15**	**Zhi Shen**	**Finger Kidney**	**0.1 cun**	**Perpenducular insertion. Use all 3 points.**
Knee joint pain	**11.05**	**Zhong Jian**	**Center Distance**	**0.2-0.3 cun**	**Perpendicular insertion. Use only one side.**
	11.13	**Dan**	**Gall Bladder**	**Micro-puncture**	**See section on micro-puncture.**
	44.06	**Jian Zhong**	**Shoulder Center**	**1.0-1.5 cun**	**Perpendicular insertion.**
	44.11	**Yun Bai**	**Cloud White**	**0.3-0.5 cun**	
	44.17	**Shui Yu**	**Water Cure**	**0.3-0.5 cun**	
	22.01	Zhong Zi	Double Son	1.0-1.5 cun	Perpendicular insertion.
	22.02	Zhong Xian	Double Saint	1.0-1.5 cun	Perpendicular insertion.
	33.12	Xin Men	Heart Gate	1.0-1.5 cun	On healthy side. Micro-puncture DT,07 to enhance the effect.
	77.09	Si Hua Zhong	4 Middle Flowers	Micro-puncture	See section on micro-puncture.
	77.11	Si Hua Xia	4 Lower Flowers	0.5-1.0 cun	Perpendicular insertion. Needle along bone.
	DT07	San Jin	Three Gold	Micro-puncture	See section on micro-puncture. Chronic knee pain
Knee pain	**11.02**	**Xiao Jian**	**Small Distance**	**0.2-0.3 cun**	**Perpendicular insertion.**
	11.16	**Huo Xi**	**Fire Knee**	**0.1 cun**	
	22.02	**Zhong Xian**	**Double Saint**	**1.0-1.5 cun**	**These are all possible combinations, do not use all points for one treatment.**
	22.15	**Xi Gai**	**Knee**	**0.5-1.0 cun**	
	44.06	**Jian Zhong**	**Shoulder Center**	**1.0-1.5 cun**	
	44.12	**Li Bai**	**Plum White**	**0.5 cun**	
	44.16	**Shang Qu**	**Upper Curve**	**0.6-1.5 cun**	
	88.25	**Zhong Jiu Li**	**Middle 9 Miles**	**0.8-2.0 cun**	
	99.03	**Huo Er**	**Fire Ear**	**0.2 cun**	**See section on micro-puncture for DT07**
	DT07	**San Jin**	**Three Gold**	**Micro-puncture**	
	22.15	**Xi Gai**	**Knee**	**0.5-1.0 cun**	**Perpendicular insertion.**
	44.06	**Jian Zhong**	**Shoulder Center**	**1.0-1.5 cun**	**Perpendicular insertion. Contra lateral. Add 44.11, 44.17.**
	99.03	**Huo Er**	**Fire Ear**	**0.2 cun**	**Mainly RA, but can treat any type of knee pain.**
	33.12	Xin Men	Heart Gate	1.0-1.5 cun	Perpendicular insertion. Contralateral
	44.06	Jian Zhong	Shoulder Center		
	88.25	Zhong Jiu Li	Middle 9 Miles	0.8-2.0 cun	Perpendicular insertion. Right side is more powerful than left side.
	1010.21	Yu Huo	Jade Fire	0.1-0.3 cun	Perpendicular insertion.
	DT07	San Jin	Three Gold	Micro-puncture	Bilaterally. See section on micro-puncture.

47

Tung Acupuncture: A Quick Reference Guide

Indications	Point #	Name Pinyin	Name English	Insertion	Comments
Knee pain cold	DT07	San Jin	Three Gold	Micro-puncture	See section on micro-puncture.
	DT07	San Jin	Three Gold	Micro-puncture	See section on micro-puncture. (Bone spur or chronic condition)
	44.06	Jian Zhong	Shoulder Center	1.0-1.5 cun	Perpendicular insertion.
	88.02	Tong Shan	Passing Mountain	0.5-0.8 cun	Perpendicular insertion.
	88.03	Tong Tian	Passing Sky	0.5-1.0 cun	
Knee pain, anterior	**11.09**	**Xin Xi**	**Heart Knee**	**0.1 cun**	**Perpendicular insertion. Use both points.** **Next to the bone.**
	11.16	**Huo Xi**	**Fire Knee**	**0.1 cun**	**Perpenducular insertion.**
	11.01	Da Jian	Big Distance Small	0.2-0.3 cun	All points perpenducular.
	11.02	Xiao Jian	Distance	0.2-0.3 cun	Apply to right side only.
	11.05	Zhong Jian	Center Distance	0.2-0.3 cun	
	22.02	Zhong Xian	Double Saint	1.0-1.5cun	Perpendicular insertion. Through from 22.05 b/c palm is more painful.
Knee spurs	77.09	Si Hua Zhong	4 Middle Flowers	Micro-puncture	See section on micro-puncture.
	77.11	Si Hua Xia	4 Lower Flowers	0.5-1.0 cun	Perpendicular insertion. Insert needle close to the Tibia. Add 33.12 to improve the therapeutic effect.
Labor difficulty	55.01	Huo Bao	Fire Bag	0.3-0.5 cun	Perpendicular insertion or micro-puncture. **Do not use on pregnant patient.**
Lack of energy	11.21	San Yan	Three Eye	0.2 cun	Perpendicular insertion. Can also add 1010.22, 22.06. If bad tempered, add 11.17.
Lacrimation due to wind exposure	77.07	San Zhong	Third Weight	1.0-2.0 cun	Needle first in prolonged cases.
	11.17	Mu	Wood	0.25 cun	Touch periosteum. Pinch point before insertion b/c painful.
	77.18	Shen Guan	Kidney Gate	0.8-2.5 cun	Perpendicular insertion. **Do not use 77.19, 77.21 on pregnant patients.**
	77.19	Di Huang	Earthly Emperor	1.0-1.5 cun	
	77.21	Ren Huang	Man Emperor	0.6-1.2 cun	
Large intestine diseases	66.05	Men Jin	Door Gold	0.5 cun	Perpendicular insertion. For male patients use left side only, for female patiens use right side. Can also Micro-puncture
	77.24	Zu Qian Jin	Foot 1000 Gold	0.5-1.0 cun	Perpendicular insertion.
	77.25	Zu Wu Jin	Foot 5 Gold	0.5-1.0 cun	
Large intestine distending pain	66.05	Men Jin	Door Gold	0.5 cun	Perpendicular insertion. Needle 66.05 first then 33.10. For 66.05: For male patients use left side only, for female patiens use right side. Can also Micro-puncture
	33.10	Chang Men	Intestine Gate		
Laryngitis	**44.07**	**Bei Mian**	**Back Face**	**0.3-0.5 cun**	**Perpendicular insertion.**
	99.07	**Er Bei**	**Ear Back**	**Micro-puncture**	**See section on micro-puncture.**
	77.24	Zu Qian Jin	Foot 1000 Gold	0.5-1.0 cun	Perpendicular insertion.
	77.25	Zu Wu Jin	Foot 5 Gold	0.5-1.0 cun	Perpendicular insertion.
	77.27	Wai San Guan	Outer 3 Gates	1.0-1.5 cun.	Perpendicular insertion. Similar to 5 tigers 11.27.
	88.09	Tong Shen	Passing Kidney	0.3-0.5 cun	Perpendicular insertion.
	88.10	Tong Wei	Passing Stomach	0.3-0.8 cun	
	88.11	Tong Bei	Passing Back	0.5-1 cun	

Tung Acupuncture: A Quick Reference Guide

Indications	Point #	Name Pinyin	Name English	Insertion	Comments
Lateral epicondylitis	77.14	**Si Hua Wai**	**4 Lateral Flowers**	**1.0-1.5 cun**	**Perpendicular insertion 28g or Micro-puncture**
Leg cramp	77.04	Bo Qiu	Catching Ball	1.0-2.0 cun	Perpendicular insertion.
Leg muscle pain	**44.07**	**Bei Mian**	Back Face	**Micro-puncture**	**See section on micro-puncture.**
	44.17	Shui Yu	Water Cure	0.3-0.5 cun	Perpendicular insertion. Add 44.06, 44.11.
Leg numbness	44.06	Jian Zhong	Shoulder Center	1.0-1.5 cun	Perpendicular insertion. Contralateral
	77.18 77.19 77.21	Shen Guan Di Huang Ren Huang	Kidney Gate Earthly Emperor Man Emperor	0.8-2.5 cun 1.0-1.5 cun 0.6-1.2 cun	Perpendicular insertion. Add these points to enhance the overall effect of the treatment. **Do not use 77.19, 77.21 on pregnant patients.**
	88.17 88.18 88.19	Zi Ma Zhong Zi Ma Shang Zi Ma Xia	Center 4 Horses Upper 4 Horses Lower 4 Horses	0.8-2.5 cun. 0.8-2.5 cun 0.8-2.5 cun	Perpendicular insertion.
	DT05	Shuang Feng	Double Phoenix	Micro-puncture	See section on micro-puncture.
Leg pain (Sorness & distending pain)	DT08	Jing Zhi	Essence Branch		Extremely good in severe cases.
Leg pain	**22.13**	**San Cha Er**	**Three Jam Two**	**1.0 – 1.5 cun**	**Towards the palm.**
	44.16	**Shang Qu**	**Upper Curve**	**0.6-1.5 cun**	**Perpendicular insertion. Contra lateral.**
	22.13 **88.27**	**San Cha Er** Xia Jiu Li	**Three Jam Two** **Lower 9 Miles**	**1.0–1.5 cun** **0.8-2.0 cun**	**22.13 towards the palm. 88.27 perpendicular insertion. Add 44.16 & 44.17 as distal points to enhance the therapeutic effect. (Anterior Tibia, shin plints, compartment syndrome)**
	22.05	Ling Gu	Androit Bone	Deep insert to 22.02	Perpendicular insertion. **Do not use on pregnant patient.**
	33.08 33.09	Shou Wu Jin Shou Qian Jin	Hand Five Gold Hand 1000 Gold	0.3-0.5 cun 0.3-0.5 cun	Perpendicular insertion.
	44.10	Tian Zong	Heaven Ancestor	1.0-1.5 cun	Perpendicular insertion. Contra lateral. Caution Biceps muscle or Cephalic vein.
	44.12	Li Bai	Plum White	0.5 cun	Perpendicular insertion.
	DT08	Jing Zhi	Essence Branch	Micro-puncture	Due to compartment syndrome. See section on micro-puncture.
	88.27	Xia Jiu Li	Lower 9 Miles	0.8-2.0 cun	Perpendicular insertion. (Due to ischemia)
Leg pain cold	44.06 88.25 88.26 88.27	Jian Zhong Zhong Jiu Li Shang Jiu Li Xia Jiu Li	Shoulder Center Middle 9 Miles Upper 9 Miles Lower 9 Miles	1.0-1.5 cun 0.8-2.0 cun 0.8-2.0 cun 0.8-2.0 cun	Perpendicular insertion.
	88.03 88.10	Tong Tian Tong Wei	Passing Sky Passing Stomach	0.5-1.0 cun 0.3-0.8 cun	Perpendicular insertion.
	DT05	Shuang Feng	Double Phoenix	Micro-puncture	See section on micro-puncture.
Leg swelling	DT08	Jing Zhi	Essence Branch	Micro-puncture	See section on micro-puncture.

49

Tung Acupuncture: A Quick Reference Guide

Indications	Point #	Name Pinyin	Name English	Insertion	Comments
Leg weakness	44.06 88.03	Jian Zhong Tong Tian	Shoulder Center Passing Sky	1.0-1.5 cun	Perpendicular insertion.
	1010.08	Zhen Jing	Tranquility	0.1-0.2 cun	Always use with 1010.01.
	1010.18	Mu Zhi	Wood Branch	0.1-0.3 cun	Perpendicular insertion. Good therapeutic effect, especially for seniors.
Leucopenia	33.11 88.14	Gan Men Qi Huang	Liver Gate This Yellow	1.0-1.5 cun 1.5-2.0 cun	Perpendicular insertion. Insert 33.11 next to the bone. **Always use left arm for 33.11.**
	66.06 66.07	Mu Liu Mu Dou	Wood Stay Wood Scoop	0.3-0.5 cun 0.3-0.5 cun	Perpendicular insertion.
Leucorrhea	11.06	Huan Chao	Return Nest	0.3 cun	Vertical insertion along bone. Either side, but not both. Leucorrhea with reddish discharge.
	33.01 33.02 33.03	Qi Men Qi Jiao Qi Zheng	This Door This Corner This Uprightness	0.2-0.5 cun 0.2-0.5 cun 0.2-0.5 cun.	Horizontal insertion. Use 3 needles total, 33.01-33.03. Insert in one side L or R. Can also Micro-puncture
	44.10 44.11	Tian Zong Yun Bai	Heaven Ancestor Cloud White	1.0-1.5 cun 0.3-0.5 cun	Perpendicular insertion. Caution Biceps muscle or Cephalic vein.
	66.02	Mu Fu	Wood Wife	0.2-0.4 cun	Perpendicular insertion. Use 30g-32g needle. Touch periosteum.
	88.09 88.10 88.11	Tong Shen Tong Wei Tong Bei	Passing Kidney Passing Stomach Passing Back	0.3-0.5 cun 0.3-0.8 cun 0.5-1.0 cun	Perpendicular insertion. Pick 2 of these 3 points (4 points at 2 thighs), Never use 3 needles same time. (Any kind of leucorrhea)
	11.24	Fu Ke	Lady Class	0.2 cun	Diagonal towards index finger. Leucorrhea with red & white discharge
	66.02 88.04 88.05 88.06	Mu Fu Jie Mei Yi Jie Mei Er Jie Mei San	Wood Wife First Sister Second Sister Third Sister	0.2-0.4 cun 1.5-2.0 cun 1.5-2.0 cun 1.5-2.0 cun	Perpendicular insertion. Always use 88.04 88.05 & 88.06 bilaterally simulGall Bladdereously. Leucorrhea with red & white discharge
Leukemia (Increased WBC)	**88.12** **88.13** **88.14**	**Ming Huang** **Tian Huang** **Qi Huang**	**Bright Yellow** **Heavenly Yellow** **This Yellow**	**1.5-2.5 cun** **1.5-2.5 cun** **1.5-2.0 cun**	**Perpendicular insertion.**
	66.06	Mu Liu	Wood Stay	0.3-0.5 cun	Perpendicular insertion.
Limbs atrophy (muscle wasting)	**66.09**	**Shui Qu**	**Water Curve**	**0.5-1.0 cun**	**Perpendicular insertion.**
Limbs weakness	66.10	Huo Lian	Fire Connection	0.5-0.8 cun	Horizontal insertion. **Use on one side only. Do not use on pregnant patient.**
Lip numbness	**VT06**	**Chun Ma**	**Lip Numbness**	**0.5 cun**	**Perpendicular.**
Lip tenderness	**77.15** **77.16**	**Shang Chun** **Xia Chun**	**Upper Lip** **Lower Lip**	**Micro-puncture** **Micro-puncture**	**Have patient bend knees to expose point.** **See section on micro-puncture.**

50

© **Theodore L. Zombolas PhD (AM), LAc, Dipl.Ac. (NCCAOM). ©**

Tung Acupuncture: A Quick Reference Guide

Indications	Point #	Name Pinyin	Name English	Insertion	Comments
Liver cirrhosis	11.20	Mu Yan	Wood Inflammation	0.2 cun	Perpendicular insertion. If bad tempered, add 11.17
	77.05 77.06 77.07	Yi Zhong Er Zhong San Zhong	First Weight Second Weight Third Weight	1.0-2.0 cun 1.0-2.0 cun 1.0-2.0 cun	Perpendicular insertion. Use all points bilaterally. 77.05 projection point of 11.14.
	88.12 88.13 88.14	Ming Huang Tian Huang Qi Huang	Bright Yellow Heavenly Yellow This Yellow	1.5-2.5 cun 1.5-2.5 cun 1.5-2.0 cun	Perpendicular insertion.
	99.02	Mu Er	Wood Ear	Just touch cartilage	
	77.29	Nei Xi Yan	Medial Eye of The Knee	1.0-1.5 cun	Perpendiculr. Bilateral.
Liver disease	66.04	Huo Zhu	Fire Master	0.3-0.8 cun	Perpendicular insertion. No moxa. Do not use on pregnant patient.
	66.06	Mu Liu	Wood Stay	0.3-0.5 cun	Perpendicular insertion.
	66.07	Mu Dou	Wood Scoop	0.3-0.5 cun	Perpendicular insertion.
	66.06	Mu Liu	Wood Stay	0.3-0.5 cun	Perpendicular insertion. Chronic Liver disease,
	88.12 88.13 88.14	Ming Huang Tian Huang Qi Huang	Bright Yellow Heavenly Yellow This Yellow	1.5-2.5 cun 1.5-2.5 cun 1.5-2.0 cun	Perpendicular insertion.
Liver disharmony	66.06 66.07	Mu Liu Mu Dou	Wood Stay Wood Scoop	0.3-0.5 cun 0.3-0.5 cun	Perpendicular insertion.
Liver GB diseases	44.16 33.11 88.12	Shang Qu Gan Men Ming Huang	Upper Curve Liver Gate Bright Yellow	Micro-puncture 1.0-1.5 cun 1.5-2.5 cun	See section on micro-puncture. Micro-puncture 44.16 first, then needle 33.11 & 88.12. Perpendicular insertion.
	77.09 77.14 88.12 88.13 88.14	Si Hua Zhong Si Hua Wai Ming Huang Tian Huang Qi Huang	4 Middle Flowers 4 Lateral Flowers Bright Yellow Heavenly Yellow This Yellow	Micro-puncture Micro-puncture 1.5-2.5 cun 1.5-2.5 cun 1.5-2.0 cun	See section on micro-puncture. Micro-puncture 77.09 & first Then perpendicular needle 88.12, 88.13 & 88.14.
Liver stagnation	66.05	Men Jin	Door Gold	0.5 cun	Perpendicular insertion. Disperse liver Stagnation & regulate Spleen. For male patients use left side only, for female patiens use right side. Can also Micro-puncture
Loin sorness	1010.22	Bi Yi	Nasal Wing	0.1-0.2 cun	Perpendicular insertion.
Loss of hearing	55.02	Hua Gu Yi	Flower Bone 1	0.5-1.0 cun	Perpendicular insertion, 30g or 32g needle. Equivalent to 22.05. Conductive type not structural change.
	88.17 88.18 88.19	Zi Ma Zhong Zi Ma Shang Zi Ma Xia	Center 4 Horses Upper 4 Horses Lower 4 Horses	0.8-2.5 cun. 0.8-2.5 cun 0.8-2.5 cun	Perpendicular insertion.
Loss of voice due to stroke	88.32	Shi Yin	Voice Loss	1.0-1.5 cun	Horizontal insertion. Bilateral. Keep knee at 90° angle and have patient swallow for induction.

51

Tung Acupuncture: A Quick Reference Guide

Indications	Point #	Name Pinyin	Name English	Insertion	Comments
Low back pain	11.15 44.13 66.12 1010.23	Zhi Shen Zhi Tong Huo San Zhou Huo	Finger Kidney Branch Through Fire Scatter Prefect Fire	0.1 cun 1.0 cun 0.5-1.0 cun 0.1-0.3 cun	Perpendicular insertion.
	11.12	Er Jiao Ming	Two Corner Bright	0.1 cun	Towards the small finger is very effective. Use both points.
	77.01 77.02	Zheng Jin Zheng Zong	Upright Tendon Uprightness Ancestry	0.5-0.8 cun 0.5-0.8 cun	Perpendicular insertion. Through the Achilles tendon. Contra lateral insertion first, then ipsi lateral insertion. Always use 77.01 with 77.02 for better results.
	22.05	Ling Gu	Androit Bone	Deep insert to 22.02	Treat in the afternoon, not morning. Good for pain in the middle of the lower back Do not use 22.05 on pregnant patient. (Acute sprain)
	22.07	Xia Bai	Lower White	0.3-0.5 cun	Needle the point under 22.03. Effective for acute lumbar sprain.
	22.04 22.05	Da Bai Ling Gu	Big White Androit Bone	Deep insert to 22.01 Deep insert to 22.02	Perpendicular insertion. Do not use on pregnant patient.
	22.04 22.05 77.21 1010.13	Da Bai Ling Gu Ren Huang Ma Jin Shui	Big White Androit Bone Man Emperor Horse Gold Water	Deep insert to 22.01 Deep insert to 22.02 0.6-1.2 cun 0.1-0.3 cun	Perpendicular insertion. Very effective combination. Adding 1010.22 will enhance the therapeutic effect. Do not use 22.04, 22.05, and 77.21 on pregnant patient.
	22.05 22.07 22.09	Ling Gu Xia Bai Wan Shun Er	Androit Bone Lower White Wrist Flow Two	Deep insert to 22.02 0.3-0.5 cun 1.0-1.5 cun	Perpendicular insertion. All effective points for low back pain. Do not use 22.05 on pregnant patient.
	22.06 22.07	Zhong Bai Xia Bai	Center White Lower White	0.3-0.5 cun 0.3-0.5 cun	Perpendicular insertion.
	22.14	San Cha San	Three Jam Three	1.0 – 1.5 cun	Towards the palm.
	77.18 77.19 77.21	Shen Guan Di Huang Ren Huang	Kidney Gate Earthly Emperor Man Emperor	0.8-2.5 cun 1.0-1.5 cun 0.6-1.2 cun	Perpendicular insertion. Do not use 77.19, 77.21 on pregnant patients.
	77.18 77.19 77.21 1010.19 1010.20	Shen Guan Di Huang Ren Huang Shui Tong Shui Jin	Kidney Gate Earthly Emperor Man Emperor Water Through Water Gold	0.8-2.5 cun 1.0-1.5 cun 0.6-1.2 cun 0.1-0.5 cun 0.1-0.5 cun	Perpendicular insertion. Add 22.06 & 22.08 to enhance the effect. Do not use 77.19, 77.21 on a pregnant patient.
	1010.19 1010.20	Shui Tong Shui Jin	Water Through Water Gold	0.1-0.5 cun 0.1-0.5 cun	Horizontal insertion. Bilateral. Sprain/strain d/t Qi blockage.
Lower abdominal pain (intestinal)	88.04 88.05 88.06	Jie Mei Yi Jie Mei Er Jie Mei San	First Sister Second Sister Third Sister	1.5-2.0 cun 1.5-2.5 cun 1.5-2.5 cun	Perpendicular insertion. Always use 3 points bilaterally.
Lower back pain due to Kidney deficiency	22.06 22.08	Zhong Bai Wan Shun Yi	Center White Wrist Flow One	0.3-0.5 cun 1.0-1.5 cun	Perpendicular insertion.
	77.18	Shen Guan	Kidney Gate	0.8-2.5 cun	Perpendicular insertion.
	1010.13 1010.14	Ma Jin Shui Ma Kuai Shui	Horse Gold Water Horse Fast Water	0.1-0.3 cun 0.1-0.3 cun	Perpendicular insertion.
	1010.19 1010.20	Shui Tong Shui Jin	Water Through Water Gold	0.1-0.5 cun 0.1-0.5 cun	Horizontal insertion. Bilateral.

Indications	Point #	Name Pinyin	Name English	Insertion	Comments
Lower extremity sprain/strain.	88.17 88.18 88.19	Zi Ma Zhong Zi Ma Shang Zi Ma Xia	Center 4 Horses Upper 4 Horses Lower 4 Horses	0.8-2.5 cun. 0.8-2.5 cun 0.8-2.5 cun	Perpendicular insertion.
Lower leg muscle pain	**11.11**	**Fei Xin**	**Lung Heart**	**0.1 cun**	**Perpendicular insertion. Use both points.**

Notes:

53

Indications	Point #	Name Pinyin	Name English	Insertion	Comments
Lumbago	11.12	Er Jiao Ming	Two Corner Bright	0.1 cun	**Use both points.**
	22.05 22.06 22.07	**Ling Gu Zhong Bai Xia Bai**	**Androit Bone Center White Lower White**	Deep insert to 22.02 0.3-0.5 cun 0.3-0.5 cun	**Perpendicular insertion. Bidirectional as needed. Do not use 22.05 on pregnant patient. Can also use 11.21, 1010.22 0.5-1.0 cun insertion. L1 – L5.**
	99.06	**Shui Er**	**Water Ear**	**0.2 cun**	**Slightly behind Nogier's cervical spine point. Confined to lumbar L2-L5.**
	1010.19 1010.20	**Shui Tong Shiu Jin**	**Water Through Water Gold**	0.1-0.5 cun 0.1-0.5 cun	Horizontal insertion. Bilateral. **Needle to the lateral side of chin. Add 77.18 to balance Kidney Y-Y. Bilaterally.**
	22.05	Ling Gu	Androit Bone	Deep insert to 22.02	Perpendicular insertion. **Do not use on pregnant patient.**
	44.02 44.03	Hou Zhui Shou Ying	Back Vertibrae Head Wisdom	0.3-0.5 cun 0.3-0.5 cun	Perpendicular insertion.
	44.17	Shui Yu	Water Cure	0.3-0.5 cun	Perpendicular insertion.
	66.09	Shui Qu	Water Curve	0.5-1.0 cun	Perpendicular insertion.
	77.03 77.04	Zheng Shi Bo Qiu	Upright Scholar Catching Ball	0.5-1.0 cun 1.0-2.0 cun	Perpendicular insertion. Through the Achilles tendon. Image popleteal - scapula.
	77.21	Ren Huang	Man Emperor	0.6-1.2 cun	Perpendicular insertion. **Do not use on pregnant patient.**
	88.09 88.10 88.11	Tong Shen Tong Wei Tong Bei	Passing Kidney Passing Stomach Passing Back	0.3-0.5 cun 0.3-0.8 cun 0.5-1.0 cun	Perpendicular insertion. Pick 2 of these 3 points (4 points at 2 thighs), Never use 3 needles same time.
	88.15 88.16	Huo Zhi Huo Quan	Fire Branch Fire Complete	1.5-2.0 cun 1.5-2.0 cun	Perpendicular insertion.
	88.17 88.18 88.19	Zi Ma Zhong Zi Ma Shang Zi Ma Xia	Center 4 Horses Upper 4 Horses Lower 4 Horses	0.8-2.5 cun. 0.8-2.5 cun 0.8-2.5 cun	Perpendicular insertion. D/t lung deficiency
	1010.02 1010.03 1010.04	Zhou Yuan Zhou Kun Zhou Lun	Prefecture Round Prefecture Elder Brother Prefecture Mountain	0.1-0.3 cun 0.1-0.3 cun 0.1-0.3 cun	Horizontal insertion.
	1010.13	Ma Jin Shui	Horse Gold Water	0.1-0.3 cun	Perpendicular insertion. Right side is more effective than left side. Use right side if patient is right handed.
	1010.23 1010.24	Zhou Huo Zhou Jin	Prefect Fire Prefect Gold	0.1-0.3 cun 0.1-0.3 cun	Perpendicular insertion.
	DT04	Wu Ling	5 Mountain Ranges	Micro-puncture	See section on micro-puncture.
	DT10	Ting Chu	Top Pillar	Micro-puncture	See section on micro-puncture.
	DT15	San Chiang	Three Rivers	Micro-puncture	See section on micro-puncture.
	L2	Shui Fu	Water Bowels	0.8-1.0 cun	Perpendicular insertion.
	77.01 77.02	Zheng Jin Zheng Zong	Upright Tendon Uprightness	0.5 – 0.8 cun	Perpendicular insertion. (Penetrate tendon more effective). Needle

54

Tung Acupuncture: A Quick Reference Guide

Indications	Point #	Name Pinyin	Name English	Insertion	Comments
Lumbago cont.			Ancestry	0.5-0.8 cun	robust patient in a sitting position; weak person with side lying position.
Lumbar sprain (Acute)	**11.12**	**Er Jiao Ming**	**Two Corner Bright**	**0.1 cun**	**Use both points.** **Do not use at same time as 1010.13.**
	11.12 **1010.13**	**Er Jiao Ming** **Ma Jin Shui**	**Two Corner Bright** **Horse Gold Water**	**Micro-puncture** **0.1 cun**	**Perpendicular insertion.** **Needle either 11.12 or 1010.13, but not both.**
	DT10	Ting Chu	Top Pillar	Micro-puncture	See section on micro-puncture.
	1010.13 1010.19	Ma Jin Shui Shui Tong	Horse Gold Water Water Through	0.1-0.3 cun 0.1-0.5 cun	Perpendicular insertion.
Lung deficiency	88.17 88.18 88.19	Zi Ma Zhong Zi Ma Shang Zi Ma Xia	Center 4 Horses Upper 4 Horses Lower 4 Horses	0.8-2.5 cun. 0.8-2.5 cun 0.8-2.5 cun	Perpendicular insertion.
Lung diseases	**22.12**	**San Cha Yi**	**Three Jam One**	**1.0 – 1.5 cun**	**Towards the palm.**
	77.24 77.25	Zu Qian Jin Zu Wu Jin	Foot 1000 Gold Foot 5 Gold	0.5-1.0 cun 0.5-1.0 cun	Perpendicular insertion.
	88.17 88.18 88.19	Zi Ma Zhong Zi Ma Shang Zi Ma Xia	Center 4 Horses Upper 4 Horses Lower 4 Horses	0.8-2.5 cun. 0.8-2.5 cun 0.8-2.5 cun	Perpendicular insertion.
	1010.19 1010.20	Shui Tong Shui Jin	Water Through Water Gold	0.1-0.5 cun 0.1-0.5 cun	Horizontal insertion. Bilateral.
Mandible pain (Difficulty opening mouth)	99.07	Er Bei	Ear Back	Micro-puncture	See section on micro-puncture.
	66.03	Hou Yin	Fire Hardness	0.3-0.5 cun	Perpendicular insertion. **Do not use on pregnant patient.**
	66.05	Men Jin	Door Gold	0.5 cun	Perpendicular insertion. For male patients use left side only, for female patiens use right side. Can also Micro-puncture
Mastitis	77.05 77.06 77.07	Yi Zhong Er Zhong San Zhong	First Weight Second Weight Third Weight	1.0-2.0 cun 1.0-2.0 cun 1.0-2.0 cun	Perpendicular insertion. Use all points bilaterally. 77.05 projection point of 11.14. (right in females)
	DT02	Fen Chi Sha	Lower Separation Branch	0.5-1.0 cun	Perpendicular insertion. Bilateral
Maxilla pain	1010.21	Yu Huo	Jade Fire	0.1-0.3 cun	Perpendicular insertion.
Meniere's Syndrome	22.05	Ling Gu	Android Bone	Deep insert to 22.02	Perpendicular insertion **Do not use 22.05 on pregnant patient.**
Meningitis (Rigidity of neck)	**66.12**	**Huo San**	**Fire Scatter**	**0.5-1.0 cun**	**Use on one side only. Always use with 66.10 & 66.11.** **Do not use on pregnant patients.**
	77.05 77.06 77.07	Yi Zhong Er Zhong San Zhong	First Weight Second Weight Third Weight	1.0-2.0 cun 1.0-2.0 cun 1.0-2.0 cun	Perpendicular insertion. Use all points bilaterally. 77.05 projection point of 11.14.
	77.07	San Zhong	Third Weight	1.0-2.0 cun	Perpendicular insertion. Dao ma. Prick first then needle 77.01. Micro-punctureting at 77.07 San Zhong may produce a better result.
Menorrhagia (Excessive menses)	11.24	Fu Ke	Lady Class	0.2 cun	Diagonal towards index finger.
	88.04 **88.05** **88.06**	**Jie Mei Yi** **Jie Mei Er** **Jie Mei San**	**First Sister** **Second Sister** **Third Sister**	**1.5-2.0 cun** **1.5-2.5 cun** **1.5-2.5 cun**	**Perpendicular insertion.** **Always use 3 points bilaterally.**

55

Indications	Point #	Name Pinyin	Name English	Insertion	Comments
Menorrhea	**22.05**	**Ling Gu**	**Android Bone**	**Deep insert to 22.02**	**Perpendicular insertion. Bidirectional as needed. Do not use on pregnant patient.**
Menorrhea hyper-Oligo	33.02	Qi Jiao	This Corner	0.2-0.5 cun	Horizontal insertion. Use 3 needles total, 33.01-33.03. Insert in one side L or R.
Menstruation irregular	L1	Shui Chung	Water Center	0.8-1.0 cun	Perpendicular insertion.
Metritis (Uterine inflammation)	66.02 66.03 66.04	Mu Fu Huo Ying Huo Zhu	Wood Wife Fire Hardness Fire Master	0.2-0.4 cun 0.3-0.5 cun 0.3-0.8 cun	Perpendicular insertion. Use 30g-32g needle. **Do not use 66.03 or 66.04 on pregnant patients.**
	66.03	Huo Ying	Fire Hardness	0.5-1.0 cun	Perpendicular insertion. **Do not use on pregnant patient.**
	66.04	Huo Zhu	Fire Master	0.3-0.8 cun	Perpendicular insertion. No moxa. **Do not use on pregnant patient.**
	66.13	Shui Jing	Water Crystal	0.5-1.0 cun	Perpendicular insertion. Unilateral or bilateral through flexor retinaculum.
	88.04 88.05 88.06	Jie Mei Yi Jie Mei Er Jie Mei San	First Sister Second Sister Third Sister	1.5-2.0 cun 1.5-2.5 cun 1.5-2.5 cun	Perpendicular insertion. Always use 3 points bilaterally.
Middle age house wife syndrome	**66.10**	**Huo Lian**	**Fire Connection**	**0.5-0.8 cun**	**Horizontal insertion. Use on one side only. Do not use on pregnant patient.**
Middle finger (Can't bend)	**66.06**	**Mu Liu**	**Wood Stay**	**0.3-0.5 cun**	**Perpendicular insertion.**
Middle finger numbness	88.01 88.02	Tong Guan Tong Shan	Penetrating Gate Passing Mountain	0.3-0.5 cun 0.5-0.8 cun	Perpendicular insertion.
Migraine	**22.05**	**Ling Gu**	**Android Bone**	**Deep insert to 22.02**	**Perpendicular insertion. Bidirectional as needed. Do not use on pregnant patient.**
	55.06 **66.08** **88.25**	**Shang Liu** **Liu Wan** **Zhong Jiu Li**	**Upper Tumor** **Sixth Finish** **Middle 9 Miles**	**0.3-0.5 cun** **0.3-0.5 cun** **0.8-2.0 cun**	**Perpendicular insertion. Deep insertion in 55.06 may result in dyspnea & discomfort. Do not use 66.08 on COPD, bronchiectasis or asthma patients.**
	66.05	**Men Jin**	**Door Gold**	**Micro-puncture**	**See section on micro-puncture. Left for males, right for females.**
	66.08	**Liu Wan**	**Sixth Finish**	**0.3-0.5 cun**	**Perpendicular insertion. Do not use with lung disease**
	77.14	**Si Hua Wai**	**4 Lateral Flowers**	**1.0-1.5 cun**	**Perpendicular insertion 28g needle or Micro-puncture**
	88.25	Zhong Jiu Li	Middle 9 Miles	0.8-2.0 cun	Perpendicular insertion. Right side is more powerful than left side.
	99.08	Er San	Ear Three	Micro-puncture	See section on micro-puncture. Do bilaterally. Add 66.08.
	1010.22	Bi Yi	Nasal Wing	0.1-0.2 cun	Perpendicular insertion.
Mitral valve disease	11.16	Huo Xi	Fire Knee	0.1 cun	Micro-puncture along spinal column region.

56

Tung Acupuncture: A Quick Reference Guide

Indications	Point #	Name Pinyin	Name English	Insertion	Comments
Mouth (Difficulty opening) mandible pain	99.07	Er Bei	Ear Back	Micro-puncture	See section on micro-puncture.
	66.03	Hou Yin	Fire Hardness	0.3-0.5 cun	Perpendicular insertion.
	66.05	Men Jin	Door Gold	0.5 cun	**Do not use 66.03 on pregnant patient.** For 66.05: For male patients use left side only, for female patiens use right side. Can also Micro-puncture
Mouth ulcer	**77.15**	**Shang Chun**	**Upper Lip**	Micro-puncture	**Have patient bend knees to expose points.**
	77.16	**Xia Chun**	**Lower Lip**	Micro-puncture	**See section on micro-puncture.**
Multiple sclerosis	**88.12**	**Ming Huang**	**Bright Yellow**	1.5-2.5 cun	**Perpendicular insertion.**
	88.13	**Tian Huang**	**Heavenly Yellow**	1.5-2.5 cun	
	88.14	**Qi Huang**	**This Yellow**	1.5-2.0 cun	
	77.18	**Shen Guan**	**Kidney Gate**	0.8-2.5 cun	**Perpendicular insertion.**
Mumps	**77.27**	Wai San Guan	**Outer 3 Gates**	1.0-1.5 cun.	**Perpendicular insertion. Similar to 5 tigers 11.27.**
Muscle spasm	**33.16**	**Qu Ling**	**Curved Mound**	0.3-0.5 cun	**Perpendicular insertion.**
Muscular atrophy Muscular dystrophy	**11.14**	Zhi San Zhong	**Finger 3 Layer**	0.1 cun	**Perpenducular insertion. Use all 3 points.** **Add 77.05 to enhance the thearaputic effect.**
Myasthenia: Eyes, difficulty opening	88.17	Zi Ma Zhong	Center 4 Horses	0.8-2.5 cun.	Perpendicular insertion. Due to deficiency of Qi.
	88.18	Zi Ma Shang	Upper 4 Horses	0.8-2.5 cun	
	88.19	Zi Ma Xia	Lower 4 Horses	0.8-2.5 cun	
Myiodesopsia	77.18	Shen Guan	Kidney Gate	0.8-2.5 cun	Perpendicular insertion.
	77.28	Guang Ming	Bright Light	0.5-1.0 cun	Use thin needle with 77.28.
Myocardial infarction	**88.01**	**Tong Guan**	**Penetrating Gate**	0.3-0.5 cun	**Perpendicular insertion.**
	88.02	**Tong Shan**	**Passing Mountain**	0.5-0.8 cun	
	77.09	**Si Hua Zhong**	**4 Middle Flowers**	2.0-3.0 cun	
	77.14	**Si Hua Wai**	**4 Lateral Flowers**	1.0-1.5 cun	
	DT11	Hou Shin	Behind Heart	Micro-puncture	See section on micro-puncture.
Myocarditis	Ear	Apex		Micro-puncture	See section on micro-puncture.
	33.12	Xin Men	Heart Gate	1.0-1.5 cun	Perpendicular insertion. Insert next to the bone. **Always use left arm.**
	77.09	Si Hua Zhong	4 Middle Flowers	Micro-puncture	See section on micro-puncture.
	77.14	Si Hua Wai	4 Lateral Flowers	1.0-1.5 cun	Perpendicular insertion.
	88.01	Tong Guan	Penetrating Gate	0.3-0.5 cun	Perpendicular insertion.
	88.02	Tong Shan	Passing Mountain	0.5-0.8 cun	
	88.03	Tong Tian	Passing Sky	0.5-1.0 cun	
Myoma of uterus	**88.06**	**Jie Mei San**	**Third Sister**	1.5-2.5 cun	**Always use 3 points bilaterally.**
Mypoia (Short sightedness)	**22.14**	**San Cha San**	**Three Jam Three**	1.0 – 1.5 cun	**Towards the palm.**
	22.07	**Xia Bai**	**Lower White**	0.3-0.5 cun	**Perpendicular insertion.**
	22.08	Wan Shun Yi	**Wrist Flow One**	1.0-1.5 cun	**Bilateral for systemic disease.**
	66.01	**Hai Bao**	**Seal**	0.1-0.3 cun	**Perpendicular insertion, contra lateral. Similar to 22.08, 22.09.**
	99.06	**Shui Er**	**Water Ear**	0.2 cun	**Add 22.08, 22.09.**
Myoplastic anemia	**11.18**	**Pi Zhong**	**Spleen Edema**	0.1 cun	**Next to bone.**

57

Tung Acupuncture: A Quick Reference Guide

Indications	Point #	Name Pinyin	Name English	Insertion	Comments
Nasal allergy	11.17	Mu	Wood	0.25 cun	Shallow insertion, but still touch periosteum. Pinch point before insertion b/c painful.
	88.17	Zi Ma Zhong	Center 4 Horses	0.8-2.5 cun.	Perpendicular insertion.
	88.18	Zi Ma Shang	Upper 4 Horses	0.8-2.5 cun	
	88.19	Zi Ma Xia	Lower 4 Horses	0.8-2.5 cun	
Nasal bleeding	44.06	Jian Zhong	Shoulder Center	1.0-1.5 cun	Perpendicular insertion. May stop bleeding immediatly.
	66.04	Hou Zhu	Fire Master	0.3-0.8 cun	Perpendicular insertion. **Do not use on pregnant patient.**
	66.08	Liu Wan	Sixth Finish	0.3-0.5 cun	Perpendicular insertion.
Nasal diseases	**88.17**	**Zi Ma Zhong**	**Center 4 Horses**	**0.8-2.5 cun**	**Perpendicular insertion. Can treat all types of nasal diseases. Mild cases need a few tx. Severe cases require more tx with longer retention.**
	88.18	**Zi Ma Shang**	**Upper 4 Horses**	**0.8-2.5 cun**	
	88.19	**Zi Ma Xia**	**Lower 4 Horses**	**0.8-2.5 cun**	
	11.07	Zhi Si Ma	Finger 4 Horse	0.1 cun	Perpendicular insertion. Use all 3 points.
	88.01	Tong Guan	Penetrating Gate	0.3-0.5 cun	Perpendicular insertion.
	88.02	Tong Shan	Passing Mountain	0.5-0.8 cun	Any of these points individually will improve the therapeutic effect.
Nasal obstruction	33.07	Hou Fu Hai	Fire Bowels	0.5-1.0 cun	Perpendicular insertion.
	44.06	Jian Zhong	Shoulder Center	1.0-1.5 cun	Perpendicular insertion. With common cold
	66.05	Men Jin	Door Gold	0.5 cun	Perpendicular insertion. For male patients use left side only, for female patiens use right side. Can also Micro-puncture
	77.22	Ce San Li	Lateral 3 Mile	0.5-1.0 cun	Perpendicular insertion. Retain the needle longer for a better effect.
Nasal pain	**55.02**	**Hua Gu Yi**	**Flower Bone 1**	**0.5-1.0 cun**	**Perpendicular insertion, 30g or 32g needle. Equivalent to 22.05.**
	11.12	Er Jiao Ming	Two Corner Bright	0.1 cun	Use both points.
Nausea	22.14	San Cha San	Three Jam Three	1.0 – 1.5 cun	Towards the palm.
Nausea & vomiting	**99.01**	**Er Huan**	**Ear Ring**	**0.2 cun**	**Insert from back to front of lobe towards root of the ear. Do not use with ear piercings.**
Neck movement restriction	**66.11**	**Huo Ju**	**Fire Chrysanthemum**	**0.5-0.8 cun**	**Horizontal insertion. Use on one side only. Do not use on pregnant patient.**

Notes:

58

Tung Acupuncture: A Quick Reference Guide

Indications	Point #	Name Pinyin	Name English	Insertion	Comments
Neck pain	11.11	Fei Xin	Lung Heart	0.1 cun	**Perpendicular insertion. Use both points.**
	44.04 44.05	Fu Ding Hou Zhi	Wealth Summit Back Branch	0.5 cun 0.3-0.7 cun	**Perpendicular insertion.**
	77.01	Zheng Jin	Upright Tendon	0.5-0.8 cun	**Perpendicular insertion. Through the Achilles tendon. Add 22.08 accessory point for neck pain. Contra lateral insertion first, then ipsi lateral insertion. Always use 77.01 with 77.02 for better results. (Herniated discs) Cervical discs C1-C7.**
	77.01 77.02	Zheng Jin Zheng Zong	Upright Tendon Uprightness Ancestry	0.5-0.8 cun 0.5-0.8 cun	**Perpendicular insertion. (All types) Add 22.08 as an accessory point.**
	77.20	Si Zhi	Four Limbs	1.0-1.5 cun	**Perpendicular insertion. Do not use on pregnant patient.**
	77.21	Ren Huang	Man Emperor	0.6-1.2 cun	Perpendicular insertion. (Acute) **Do not use on pregnant patient.**
	1010.07	Zong Shu	Total Pivot	0.1-0.2 cun	Insert downward. Most effective with Micro-punctureting with extreme caution.
	DT17	Chong Xiao	Expanding Heaven	Micro-puncture	See section on micro-puncture.
Neck sprain	22.01	Zhong Zi	Double Son	1.0-1.5 cun	Perpendicular insertion. May only need a single treatment.
	22.03 22.06	Shang Bai Zhong Bai	Upper White Center White	0.3-0.5 cun 0.3-0.5 cun	Perpendicular insertion.
	22.14	San Cha San	Three Jam Three	1.0-1.5 cun	Towards the palm.
Needle shock	88.25	Zhong Jiu Li	Middle 9 Miles	0.8-2.0 cun	Perpendicular insertion.

Notes:

59

Indications	Point #	Name Pinyin	Name English	Insertion	Comments
Nephritis	22.06	Zhong Bai	Center White	0.3-0.5 cun	Perpendicular insertion.
	22.07	Xia Bai	Lower White	0.3-0.5 cun	
	22.08	Wan Shun Yi	Wrist Flow One	1.0-1.5 cun	Perpendicular insertion. (Esp. for female but only needle one hand). (Acute or chronic)
	22.09	Wan Shun Er	Wrist Flow Two	1.0-1.5 cun	
	44.02	Hou Zhui	Back Vertibrae	0.3-0.5 cun	Perpendicular insertion. (HTN)
	44.03	Shou Ying	Head Wisdom	0.3-0.5 cun	
	44.17	Shui Yu	Water Cure	Micro-puncture	To produce yellow fluid. See section on micro-puncture. (Protein urea)
	66.14	Shui Xiang	Water Phase	0. 3-.05 cun	Perpendicular insertion. Through anterior margin of the tendon. Insertion through flexor tetinaculum.
	66.15	Shui Xian	Water Fairy	0.5 cun	
	88.09	Tong Shen	Passing Kidney	0.3-0.5 cun	Perpendicular insertion.
	88.10	Tong Wei	Passing Stomach	0.3-0.8 cun	
	88.11	Tong Bei	Passing Back	0.5-1.0 cun	
	1010.13	Ma Jin Shui	Horse Gold Water	0.1-0.3 cun	Perpendicular insertion. Right side is more effective than left side. Use right side if patient is right handed.
	L1	Shui Chung	Water Center	0.8-1.0 cun	Perpendicular insertion.
	L2	Shui Fu	Water Bowels	0.8-1.0 cun	
	VT05	Fu Chao 23	Bowel Nest 23	Micro-puncture	See section on micro-puncture.
	L2	Shui Fu	Water Bowels	0.8-1.0 cun	Perpendicular insertion. Acute
Nephrolithiasis (Kidney stone)	1010.13	Ma Jin Shui	Horse Gold Water	0.1-0.3 cun	Perpendicular insertion. Right side is more effective than left side. Use right side if patient is right handed.
Nephrosis	22.06	Zhong Bai	Center White	0.3-0.5 cun	Perpendicular insertion.
	22.07	Xia Bai	Lower White	0.3-0.5 cun	
	22.07	Xia Bai	Lower White	0.3-0.5 cun	Perpendicular insertion.
Nerve impingement	33.08	Shou Wu Jin	Hand Five Gold	0.3-0.5 cun	Perpendicular insertion.
	33.09	Shou Qian Jin	Hand Thousand Gold	0.3-0.5 cun	
Nervousness	66.04	Huo Zhu	Fire Master	0.3-0.8 cun	Perpendicular insertion. No moxa. Do not use on pregnant patient.
	99.04	Tu Er	Earth Ear	0.2 cun	
	1010.05	Qian Hui	Anterior Meeting	0.1-0.3 cun	Insertion anterior to posterior. Between 1010.01 & 1010.08. (Psychoneurosis)
Neuralgia	33.08	Shou Wu Jin	Hand Five Gold	0.3-0.5 cun	Perpendicular insertion.
	33.09	Shou Qian Jin	Hand 1000 Gold	0.3-0.5 cun	
Neurosis	33.14	Di Shi	Earth Scholar	1.0-1.5 cun	Perpendicular insertion.
	99.04	Tu Er	Earth Ear	0.2 cun	Hysteria nervousness, psychoneurosys.
Nocturnal crying (child)	11.13	Dan	Gall Bladder	Micro-puncture	See section on micro-puncture.
	1010.08	Zhen Jing	Tranquility	0.1-0.2 cun	Insert towards nose. Always use with 1010.01.
Nocturnal shock (Nightmares)	88.12	Ming Huang	Bright Yellow	1.5-2.5 cun	Perpendicular insertion. Improves in 3 weeks.
	88.13	Tian Huang	Heavenly Yellow	1.5-2.5 cun	
	88.14	Qi Huang	This Yellow	1.5-2.0 cun	
Nose bleed	44.06	Jian Zhong	Shoulder Center	1.0-1.5 cun	Perpendicular insertion. Add 22.09. Middle of deltoid muscle.

Tung Acupuncture: A Quick Reference Guide

Indications	Point #	Name Pinyin	Name English	Insertion	Comments
Nose dryness	**88.17** **88.18** **88.19**	**Zi Ma Zhong** **Zi Ma Shang** **Zi Ma Xia**	**Center 4 Horses** **Upper 4 Horses** **Lower 4 Horses**	**0.8-2.5 cun.** **0.8-2.5 cun** **0.8-2.5 cun**	**Perpendicular insertion. Treats all types of nasal diseases. Mild cases require a few Tx. Severe cases require more Tx with longer retention.**
Nose, running	11.17	Mu	Wood	0.25 cun	Shallow insertion, but still touch periosteum. Pinch point before insertion b/c painful.
Numbess of the hand	66.11	Huo Ju	Fire Chrysanthemum	0.5-0.8 cun	Horizontal insertion. **Do not use on pregnant patient.**
	77.22 77.23	Ce San Li Ce Xia San Li	Lateral 3 Mile Below Lateral 3 Mile	0.5-1.0 cun 0.5-1.0 cun	Perpendicular insertion. Ipsilateral treatment.
Numbness in extremites	DT05	Shuang Feng	Double Phoenix	Micro-puncture	See section on micro-puncture.
Numbness of middle finger	88.01 88.02	Tong Guan Tong Shan	Penetrating Gate Passing Mountain	0.3-0.5 cun 0.5-0.8 cun	Perpendicular insertion.
Obesity	**88.09** **88.10** **88.11**	**Tong Shen** **Tong Wei** **Tong Bei**	**Passing Kidney** **Passing Stomach** **Passing Back**	**0.3-0.5 cun** **0.3-0.8 cun** **0.5-1.0 cun**	**Perpendicular insertion. Excessive water or fat retention. (For slimming effect)**
	77.14	Si Hua Wai	4 Lateral Flowers	Micro-puncture	See section on micro-puncture.
	77.27	Wai San Guan	Outer 3 Gates	Micro-puncture	Micro-punture at 77.09 also to enhance the therapeutic effect.
	88.12	Ming Huang	Bright Yellow	1.5-2.5 cun	Perpendicular insertion.
Occipitalgia	11.07	Zhi Si Ma	Finger 4 Horse	0.1 cun	Perpendicular insertion. Use all 3 points.
Occiput pain.	77.01 77.02	Zheng Jin Zheng Zong	Upright Tendon Uprightness Ancestry	0.5-0.8 cun 0.5-0.8 cun	Perpendicular insertion. (Penetrate tendon more effective). Needle robust patient in a sitting position; weak person with side lying position.
Oligo menorrhea	11.24	Fu Ke	Lady Class	0.2 cun	Diagonal towards index finger.
Oligoptyalism (Dry mouth) (DM)	88.09 88.10 88.11	Tong Shen Tong Wei Tong Bei	Passing Kidney Passing Stomach Passing Back	0.3-0.5 cun 0.3-0.8 cun 0.5-1.0 cun	Perpendicular insertion.
Opthalmalgia	77.09 77.10	Si Hua Zhong Si Hua Fu	4 Middle Flowers 4 Append Flowers	2.0-3.0 cun Micro-puncture	Perpendicular insertion. See section on micro-puncture. 28g needle. Right side has stronger effect.
	88.12 88.13 88.14	Ming Huang Tian Huang Qi Huang	Bright Yellow Heavenly Yellow This Yellow	1.5-2.5 cun 1.5-2.5 cun 1.5-2.0 cun	Perpendicular insertion. Bilateral.
	55.02	Hua Gu Yi	Flower Bone 1	0.5-1.0 cun	Perpendicular insertion, 30g or 32g needle. Equivalent to 22.05.
	11.01 11.02	Da Jian Xiao Jian	Big Distance Small Distance	0.2-0.3 cun 0.2-0.3 cun	All points perpenducular.
Optic atrophy	77.18 77.28	Shen Guan Guang Ming	Kidney Gate Bright Light	0.8-2.5 cun 0.5-1.0 cun	Perpendicular insertion. Use thin needle with 77.28.

61

Tung Acupuncture: A Quick Reference Guide

Indications	Point #	Name Pinyin	Name English	Insertion	Comments
Oral ulceration	Ear	Apex		Micro-puncture	See section on micro-puncture.
	77.08	Si Hua Shang	4 Upper Flowers	2.0-3.0 cun	Perpendicular insertion.
	77.09	Si Hua Zhong	4 Middle Flowers	Micro-puncture	
	77.15	Shang Chun	Upper Lip	Micro-puncture	Have patient bend knees to expose
	77.16	Xia Chun	Lower Lip	Micro-puncture	point. See section on micro-puncture.
Osteoarthritis	**22.06**	**Zhong Bai**	**Center White**	**0.3-0.5 cun**	**Perpendicular insertion.**
	22.07	**Xia Bai**	**Lower White**	**0.3-0.5 cun**	**Can also use 11.21, 1010.22 in place of 22.06**
	11.27	Wu Hu	Five Tigers	0.2 cun	Perpendicular insertion. Lower body pain, ie. Feet. Use up to 3 needles.
	88.14	Qi Huang	This Yellow	1.5-2.0 cun	Perpendicular insertion.
Otitis media	**77.14**	**Si Hua Wai**	**4 Lateral Flowers**	**Micro-puncture**	**See section on micro-puncture. Chronic in children**
	11.26	Zhi Wu	Control Dirt	Micro-puncture	See section on micro-puncture.
	77.22	Ce San Li	Lateral 3 Mile	Micro-puncture	See section on micro-puncture.
	77.23	Ce Xia San Li	Below Lateral 3 Mile	0.5-1.0 cun	Perpendicular insertion.
Ovarian duct obstruction	11.06	Huan Chao	Return Nest	0.3 cun	Vertical insertion along bone. Either side, but not both. Use with 11.24 for better therapeutic effect.
	11.24	Fu Ke	Lady Class	0.2 cun	Diagonal towards index finger.
Pain along Shaoyang channel	**88.25**	**Zhong Jiu Li**	**Middle 9 Miles**	**0.8-2.0 cun**	**Perpendicular insertion. All types of pain of the Shaoyang channel.**
Pain chronic (Any type)	**1010.01**	**Zheng Hui**	**Uprightness Meeting**	**0.1-0.3 cun**	**Horizontal insertion.**
	1010.08	**Zhen Jing**	**Tranquility**	**0.1-0.2 cun**	
Pain in extremities	DT05	Shuang Feng	Double Phoenix	Micro-puncture	See section on micro-puncture.
Pain in hands and feet	66.04	Huo Zhu	Fire Master	0.3-0.8 cun	Perpendicular insertion. No moxa. **Do not use on pregnant patient.**
Pain in the heel	**11.27**	**Wu Hu**	**Five Tigers**	**0.2 cun**	**Perpendicular insertion. Needle all 5 points**
	22.05	**Lin Gu**	**Android Bone**	**Deep insert to 22.02**	Perpendicular insertion. **Needle along the bone. Do not use on pregnant patient.**
	22.07	**Xia Bai**	**Lower White**	**0.3-0.5 cun**	Perpendicular insertion.
	1010.06	**Hou Hui**	**Posterior Meetings**	**0.1-0.3 cun**	**Horizontal.**
	77.09	Si Hua Zhong	4 Middle Flowers	Micro-puncture	See section on micro-puncture.
	77.11	Si Hua Xia	4 Lower Flowers	0.5-1.0 cun	Perpendicular insertion. Along the bone.
Pain in whole body	**88.04**	**Jie Mei Yi**	**First Sister**	**1.5-2.0 cun**	**Perpendicular insertion.**
Pain of legs	DT08	Jing Zhi	Essence Branch	Micro-puncture	Due to compartment syndrome
Pain of the acromion	22.01	Zhong Zi	Double Son	1.0-1.5 cun	Perpendicular insertion.
	22.02	Zhong Xian	Double Saint	1.0-1.5 cun	
Pain of the acromion	88.09	Tong Shen	Passing Kidney	0.3-0.5 cun	Perpendicular insertion.
	88.10	Tong Wei	Passing Stomach	0.3-0.8 cun	
	88.11	Tong Bei	Passing Back	0.5-1.0 cun	

Tung Acupuncture: A Quick Reference Guide

Indications	Point #	Name Pinyin	Name English	Insertion	Comments
Pain of the acromion	88.25	Zhong Jiu Li	Middle 9 Miles	0.8-2.0 cun	Perpendicular insertion.
	88.26	Shang Jiu Li	Upper 9 Miles	0.8-2.0 cun	
	88.27	Xia Jiu Li	Lower 9 Miles	0.8-2.0 cun	
	77.23	Ce Xia San Li	Below Lateral 3 Mile	0.5-1.0 cun	
Pain of the finger joints	11.27	Wu Hu	Five Tigers	0.2 cun	Perpendicular insertion.
	33.13	Ren Shi	Human Scholar	0.5-1.0 cun	Perpendicular insertion.
Pain of the thigh	22.14	San Cha San	Three Jam Three	1.0 – 1.5 cun	Towards the palm.
	22.14	San Cha San	Three Jam Three	1.0 – 1.5 cun	22.14 towards the palm.
	88.26	Shang Jiu Li	Upper 9 Miles	0.8-2.0 cun	88.26 perpendiculars.
	88.25	Zhong Jiu Li	Middle 9 Miles	0.8-2.0 cun	Perpendicular insertion.
	88.26	Shang Jiu Li	Upper 9 Miles	0.8-2.0 cun	
	88.27	Xia Jiu Li	Lower 9 Miles	0.8-2.0 cun	
	DT.09	Jin Lin	Gold Forest	Micro-puncture	See section on micro-puncture.
Pain of the wrist joint	22.08	Wan shun Yi	Wrist Flow One	1.0-1.5 cun	Perpendicular insertion.
	22.09	Wan Shun Er	Wrist Flow Two	1.0-1.5 cun	
	77.22	Ce San Li	Lateral 3 Mile	0.5-1.0 cun	Perpendicular insertion. Ipsilateral.
	77.22	Ce San Li	Lateral 3 Mile	0.5-1.0 cun	Perpendicular insertion.
	77.23	Ce Xia San Li	Below Lateral 3 Mile	0.5-1.0 cun	
Pain of uterus (Acute or chronic)	11.24	Fu Ke	Lady Class	0.2 cun	Diagonal towards index finger.
Palm pain	**33.13**	**Ren Shi**	**Human Scholar**	**0.5-1.0 cun**	**Perpendicular insertion.**

Notes:

Indications	Point #	Name Pinyin	Name English	Insertion	Comments
Palpitations	11.13	Dan	Gall Bladder	Micro-puncture	See section on micro-puncture.
	33.04	Huo Chuan	Fire Threaded	0.3-0.5 cun	Perpendicular insertion.
	33.12	Xin Men	Heart Gate	1.0-1.5 cun	Heart Gate. Always use left arm. CW twist: for intestinal pain, CCW twist: for chest tension. Insertion next to the bone.
	33.16	Qu Ling	Curved Mound	Micro-puncture	See section on micro-puncture.
	66.03	Huo Ying	Fire Hardness	0.3-0.5 cun	Perpendicular insertion. Do not use on pregnant patient.
	88.01	Tong Guan	Penetrating Gate	0.3-0.5 cun	Perpendicular insertion.
	88.02	Tong Shan	Passing Mountain	0.5-0.8 cun	Perpendicular insertion.
	88.03	Tong Tian	Passing Sky	0.5-1.0 cun	Perpendicular insertion.
	Ear	Apex		Micro-puncture	See section on micro-puncture.
	11.02 11.05	Xiao Jian Zhong Jian	Small Distance Center Distance	0.2-0.3 cun 0.2-0.3 cun	Perpendicular insertion. Apply to right side. 11.05 is mostly used for this condition.
	11.19	Xin Chang	Heart Normal	0.1-0.2 cun	Perpendicular insertion, use both points.
	22.14	San Cha San	Three Jam Three	1.0 – 1.5 cun	Towards the palm.
	66.10	Huo Lian	Fire Connection	0.5-0.8 cun	Horizontal insertion. Only use one point per treatment. Do not use on pregnant patient.
	66.11	Huo Ju	Fire Chrysanthemum	0.5-0.8 cun	Horizontal insertion. Use on one side only. Do not use on pregnant patient.
	77.08	Si Hua Shang	4 Upper Flowers	3.0-3.5 cun	Perpendicular insertion.
	77.13	Si Hua Li	4 Inner Flowers	1.5-2.0 cun	Perpendicular insertion.
	88.01 88.02 88.03	Tong Guan Tong Shan Tong Tian	Penetrating Gate Passing Mountain Passing Sky	0.3-0.5 cun 0.5-0.8 cun 0.5-1.0 cun	Perpendicular insertion. Only pick one or two points on one leg per treatment.
	88.29 88.30	Nei Tong Guan Nei Tong Shan	Inner Passing Gate Inner Passing Mountain	1.0 cun 1.0 cun	Perpendicular insertion.
	88.31	Nei Tong Tian	Inner Passing Sky	1.0 cun	Perpendicular insertion.
	99.03	Huo Er	Fire Ear	0.2 cun	
	1010.07	Zong Shu	Total Pivot	0.1-0.2 cun	Insert downward. Most effective with Micro-punctureting with extreme caution.
	1010.23	Zhou Huo	Prefect Fire	0.1-0.3 cun	Perpendicular insertion.
	VT04	Wei Mao Chi	Stomach Hair 7	Micro-puncture	See section on micro-puncture.
Palsy	55.06	Shang Liu	Upper Tumor	0.3-0.5 cun	Perpendicular insertion. Do not make deep insertion = dyspnea & discomfort.
Panacea for diseases	22.16	Wan Bing	10,000 Maladies	0.5 cun	Perpendicular.
Paraesthesia	88.01 88.02 88.03	Tong Guan Tong Shan Tong Tian	Penetrating Gate Passing Mountain Passing Sky	0.3-0.5 cun 0.5-0.8 cun 0.5-1.0 cun	Perpendicular insertion.
Paralysis Lower limb	1010.25	Zhou Shui	Prefect Water	0.1-0.3 cun	Insert upward or downward, use 2 needles.

64

Tung Acupuncture: A Quick Reference Guide

Indications	Point #	Name Pinyin	Name English	Insertion	Comments
Parathyroiditis	88.32	Shi Yin	Voice Loss	1.0-1.5 cun	Horizontal insertion. Bilateral. Keep knee at 90° angle and have patient swallow for induction.
Parkinson's disease	77.18 77.19 77.21 88.26 88.27 88.12 88.13 88.14 1010.05 1010.06	Shen Guan Di Huang Ren Huang Shang Jiu Li Xia Jiu Li Ming Huang Tian Huang Qi Huang Qian Hui Hou Hui	Kidney Gate Earthly Emperor Man Emperor Upper 9 Miles Lower 9 Miles Bright Yellow Heavenly Yellow This Yellow Anterior Meeting Posterior Meetings	0.8-2.5 cun 1.0-1.5 cun 0.6-1.2 cun 0.8-2.0 cun 0.8-2.0 cun 1.5-2.5 cun 1.5-2.5 cun 1.5-2.0 cun 0.1-0.3 cun 0.1-0.3 cun	In treating Parkinson's, you must needle groups alternating between: (1010.05, 1010.06) (88.26, 88.27) (88.12, 88.13, 88.14, 77.18, 77.19, 77.21) Perpendicuar insertion. To improve effect, add scalp acupuncture or 4 gates. Do not use 77.19, 77.21 on pregnant patient.
	1010.01	Zheng Hui	Uprightness Meeting	0.1-0.3 cun	Horizontal insertion. Add 1010.08. Angle and direction of insertion is anterior to posterior insert 60°-90°.
	77.18 88.12	Shen Guan Ming Huang	Kidney Gate Bright Yellow	0.8-2.5 cun 1.5-2.5 cun	Perpendicular insertion.
	77.18 88.12 88.14	Shen Guan Ming Huang Qi Huang	Kidney Gate Bright Yellow This Yellow	0.8-2.5 cun 1.5-2.5 cun 1.5-2.5 cun	Perpendicular insertion.
	1010.01 1010.05 1010.18	Zheng Hui Qian Hui Mu Zhi	Uprightness Meeting Anterior Meeting Wood Branch	0.1-0.3 cun 0.1-0.3 cun 0.1-0.3 cun	Horizontal insertion.
Pelvic congestion syndrome	66.13	Shui Jing	Water Crystal	0.5-1.0 cun	Perpendicular insertion unilateral or bilateral.
Pelvic infloamatory disease	66.13	Shui Jing	Water Crystal	0.5-1.0 cun	Perpendicular insertion unilateral or bilateral.
Pelvic pain	66.13	Shui Jing	Water Crystal	0.5-1.0 cun	Perpendicular insertion unilateral or bilateral.
Peptic ulcer	66.04	Huo Zhu	Fire Master	0.3-0.8 cun	Perpendicular insertion. Do not use on pregnant patients.
	88.04	Jie Mei Yi	First Sister	1.5-2.0 cun	Perpendicular insertion. complications (Esp. hemorrhage)
Pericarditis	88.01 88.02 88.03	Tong Guan Tong Shan Tong Tian	Penetrating Gate Passing Mountain Passing Sky	0.3-0.5 cun 0.5-0.8 cun 0.5-1.0 cun	Perpendicular insertion. Only pick one or two points on one leg per treatment.
Periductal mastitis	11.14	Zhi San Zhong	Finger 3 Layer	0.1 cun	Perpenducular insertion. Use all 3 points. Add 77.05 to enhance the thearaputic effect.
Peripheral edema	44.08	Ren Zong	Man Ancestor	0.8 cun	Perpendicular insertion. (K failure) Caution Biceps muscle or Cephalic vein.
	66.09	Shui Qu	Water Curve	0.5-1.0 cun	Perpendicular insertion.
Peritonsillar abscess	77.24 77.25	Zu Qian Jin Zu Wu Jin	Foot 1000 Gold Foot 5 Gold	0.5-1.0 cun 0.5-1.0 cun	Perpendicular insertion.
Periumbilical pain	VT05	Fu Chao 23	Bowel Nest 23	Micro-puncture	See section on micro-puncture.

65

Tung Acupuncture: A Quick Reference Guide

Indications	Point #	Name Pinyin	Name English	Insertion	Comments
Persisted carbuncles	11.26	Zhi Wu	Control Dirt	Micro-puncture	See section on micro-puncture.
Phalangitis	**22.11**	**Tu Shui**	**Earth Water**	**0.2-0.3 cun**	**Perpendicular insertion. Not due to arthritis.**
Phantom pain	**1010.01** **1010.08**	**Zheng Hui** **Zhen Jing**	**Uprightness Meeting** **Tranquility**	 **0.1-0.3 cun** **0.1-0.2 cun**	**Horizontal insertion.**
Pharyngitis	1010.22	Bi Yi	Nasal Wing	0.1-0.2 cun	Perpendicular insertion..
Photophobia	**55.02**	**Hua Gu Yi**	**Flower Bone 1**	**0.5-1.0 cun**	**Perpendicular insertion, 30g or 32g needle. Equivalent to 22.05.**
Placenta accreta (retention)	**66.03**	**Huo Ying**	**Fire Hardness**	**0.3-0.5 cun**	**Perpendicular insertion.** **Do not use on pregnant patient.**
	55.01	Huo Bao	Fire Bag	0.3-0.5 cun	Perpendicular insertion or micro-puncture. **Do not use on pregnant patient.**
Placental dystocia	66.03	Huo Ying	Fire Hardness	0.3-0.5 cun	Perpendicular insertion. **Do not use on pregnant patient.**
Pleurisy	77.09	Si Hua Zhong	4 Middle Flowers	Micro-punture	See section on micro-puncture.
	88.17 88.18 88.19	Zi Ma Zhong Zi Ma Shang Zi Ma Xia	Center 4 Horses Upper 4 Horses Lower 4 Horses	0.8-2.5 cun. 0.8-2.5 cun 0.8-2.5 cun	Perpendicular insertion.
Pleuritis	**77.26**	**Qi Hu**	**Seven Tigers**	**0.5-0.8 cun**	**Perpendicular insertion. Use all 3 points at same time contra lateral. (Pneumonia or infectious disease) Similar to 5 tigers 11.27.**
	11.07	Zhi Si Ma	Finger 4 Horse	0.1 cun	Perpendicular insertion. Use all 3 points.
	77.09 88.17 88.18 88.19	Si Hua Zhong Zi Ma Zhong Zi Ma Shang Zi Ma Xia	4 Middle Flowers Center 4 Horses Upper 4 Horses Lower 4 Horses	Micro-puncture 0.8-2.5 cun 0.8-2.5 cun 0.8-2.5 cun	See section on micro-puncture. Perpendicular insertion. Micro-puncture 77.09 first, then needle the rest of the points.
Pneumonia	22.01	Zhong Zi	Double Son	1.0-1.5 cun	Perpendicular insertion.
	22.01 22.02	Zhong Zi Zhong Xian	Double Son Double Saint	1.0-1.5cun 1.0-1.5 cun	Perpendicular insertion. Through from 22.05 b/c palm is more painful.
	22.02	Zhong Xian	Double Saint	1.0-1.5 cun	Perpendicular insertion.
	22.04	Da Bai	Big White	Micro-puncture	See section on micro-puncture. **Do not use on pregnant patients.**
	22.11	Tu Shui	Earth Water	0.2-0.3 cun	Perpendicular insertion.
	33.16	Qu Ling	Curved Mound	Micro-puncture	See section on micro-puncture.
Poliomyelitis	**44.12**	**Li Bai**	**Plum White**	**0.5 cun**	**Perpendicular insertion. (Lower extremities muscle wasting)**
	44.15 **44.16**	**Xia Qu** **Shang Qu**	**Lower Curve** **Upper Curve**	**0.6-1.0 cun** **0.6-1.5 cun**	**Perpendicular insertion.**
	66.06 **66.07**	**Mu Liu** **Mu Dou**	**Wood Stay** **Wood Scoop**	**0.3-0.5 cun** **0.3-0.5 cun**	**Perpendicular insertion.** **Strengthen muscle tone**
	44.06	**Jian Zhong**	**Shoulder Center**	**0.5-1.0 cun**	**Perpendicular insertion.** **(Infantile paralysis)**
	44.10 44.11	Tian Zong Yun Bai	Heaven Ancestor Cloud White	1.0-1.5 cun 0.3-0.5 cun	Perpendicular insertion. Caution Biceps muscle or Cephalic vein. (Muscle atrophy) Add 44.06, 44.17.
Pollen allergies	88.17 88.18 88.19	Zi Ma Zhong Zi Ma Shang Zi Ma Xia	Center 4 Horses Upper 4 Horses Lower 4 Horses	0.8-2.5 cun. 0.8-2.5 cun 0.8-2.5 cun	Perpendicular insertion. Needle 88.17 first.

Tung Acupuncture: A Quick Reference Guide

Indications	Point #	Name Pinyin	Name English	Insertion	Comments
Polyuria	**11.06**	**Huan Chao**	**Return Nest**	**0.3 cun**	**Vertical insertion along bone. Either side, but not both.**
	22.05	**Ling Gu**	**Androit Bone**	**Deep insert to 22.02**	**Perpendicular insertion. Bidirectional as needed. Increased frequency, bladder infection. Do not use on pregnant patient.**
	1010.14	Ma Kuai Shui	Horse Fast Water	0.1-0.3 cun	Perpendicular insertion.
Poor appetite	22.05	Ling Gu	Androit Bone	Deep insert to 22.02	Perpendicular insertion. **Do not use on pregnant patient.**
	66.05	Men Jin	Door Gold	0.5 cun	Perpendicular insertion. For male patients use left side only, for female patiens use right side. Can also Micro-puncture
	77.08	Si Hua Shang	4 Upper Flowers	2.0-3.0 cun	Perpendicular insertion.
Poor wound healing	11.26	Zhi Wu	Control Dirt	Micro-puncture	Needle for cuts on upper extremity. See section on micro-puncture.
Preeclampsia	**66.14** **66.15**	**Shui Xiang** **Shui Xian**	**Water Phase** **Water Fairy**	**0.3-05 cun** **0.5 cun**	**Perpendicular insertion. Through anterior margin of the tendon. Insertion through flexor tetinaculum.**
Premature ejaculation	**11.15**	**Zhi Shen**	**Finger Kidney**	**0.1 cun**	**Perpenducular insertion. Use all 3 points.**
	77.18	**Shen Guan**	**Kidney Gate**	0.8-2.5 cun	Perpendicular insertion.
	77.18 **77.19** **77.21**	**Shen Guan** **Di Huang** **Ren Huang**	**Kidney Gate** **Earthly Emperor** **Man Emperor**	**0.8-2.5 cun** **1.0-1.5 cun** **0.6-1.2 cun**	**Perpendicular insertion. Add 1010.19, 1010.20 for a better therapeutic effect. Do not use 77.19, 77.21 on pregnant patients.**
	77.18	Shen Guan	Kidney Gate	1.5-2.0 cun	Perpendicular insertion.
	77.19 77.21	Di Huang Ren Huang	Earthly Emperor Man Emperor	1.0-1.5 cun 0.6-1.2 cun	Perpendicular insertion. **Do not use these points on pregnant patient.**
	88.09 88.10 88.11	Tong Shen Tong Wei Tong Bei	Passing Kidney Passing Stomach Passing Back	0.3-0.5 cun 0.3-0.8 cun 0.5-1.0 cun	Perpendicular insertion. Pick 2 of these 3 points (4 points at 2 thighs), Never use 3 needles same time. Help prevent miscarriage.
Premenstrual tension syndrome	11.24	Fu Ke	Lady Class	0.2 cun	Diagonal towards index finger.
Proctitis (Rectum)	33.10	Chang Men	Intestine Gate	1.0-1.5 cun	Perpendicular insertion. Insert 33.10 next to the bone. **Always use left arm.**
Prostatitis	77.08 77.17	Si Huan Sang Tian Huang	4 Upper Flowers Heaven Emperor	2.0-3.0 cun 0.5-1.0 cun	These points will provide exceptional results. Add 66.04 along the bone to enhance the therapeutic effect.
Protein urea	44.17	Shui Yu	Water Cure	Micro-puncture	See section on micro-puncture.

Notes:

Tung Acupuncture: A Quick Reference Guide

Indications	Point #	Name Pinyin	Name English	Insertion	Comments
Pruritis	**11.17**	**Mu**	Wood	**0.25 cun**	**Pinch point before insertion b/c painful. Shallow insertion, but still touch periosteum.**
	88.17 **88.18** **88.19**	**Zi Ma Zhong** **Zi Ma Shang** **Zi Ma Xia**	**Center 4 Horses** **Upper 4 Horses** **Lower 4 Horses**	**0.8-2.5 cun.** **0.8-2.5 cun** **0.8-2.5 cun**	**Perpendicular insertion. (Itching)**
	DT01 DT02	Fen Chi Shang Fen Chi Sha	Upper Separation Branch Lower Separation Branch	1.0-1.5 cun 0.5-1.0 cun	Perpendicular insertion. Bilateral
Psoriasis	**88.17** **88.18** **88.19**	**Zi Ma Zhong** **Zi Ma Shang** **Zi Ma Xia**	**Center 4 Horses** **Upper 4 Horses** **Lower 4 Horses**	**0.8-2.5 cun.** **0.8-2.5 cun** **0.8-2.5 cun**	**Perpendicular insertion.** **Give Vit C 2000mg, B complex vitamins,. Zinc 50mg,**
	99.07	Er Bei	Ear Back	Micro-puncture	Treat once a week. See section on micro-puncture.
Psychosis (Paranoid type)	**1010.12**	**Zheng Ben**	**Upright Source**	**0.1-0.2 cun**	**Hearing/visual hallucinations.**
Ptosis	77.28	**Guang Ming**	**Bright Light**	**0.5-1.0 cun**	**Perpendicular insertion. Use thinner needle 30g. Eyes open in 3 sessions.**
	66.05 66.11	Men Jin Hou Ju	Door Gold Fire Chrysanthemum	0.5 cun 0.5-0.8 cun	**Do not use 66.11 on pregnant patient.** For 66.05: For male patients use left side only, for female patiens use right side. Can also Micro-puncture. (Due to myasthenia)
Ptyalism	11.25	Zhi Xian	Stop Saliva	0.2 cun	Perpendicular insertion.
Pudendum swelling	11.06	Huan Chao	Return Nest	0.3 cun	Vertical insertion along bone. Either side, but not both.
	11.24	Fu Ke	Lady Class	0.2 cun	Diagonal towards index finger.
	66.03 66.04	Huo Ying Huo Zhu	Fire Hardness Fire Master	0.3-0.5 cun 0.3-0.8 cun	Perpendicular insertion. These points can also be used for this condition. **Do not use on pregnant patient.**
Pulmonary tuberculosis	88.17 88.18 88.19	Zi Ma Zhong Zi Ma Shang Zi Ma Xia	Center 4 Horses Upper 4 Horses Lower 4 Horses	0.8-2.5 cun. 0.8-2.5 cun 0.8-2.5 cun	Perpendicular insertion.
Purpuras	55.05	Hua Gu Si	Flower Bone 4	0.5-1.0 cun	Perpendicular insertion.
Qi & Blood disorders	88.28	Jie	Release Point	0.3-0.5 cun	Perpendicular insertion.
Qi deficiency	22.05	Ling Gu	Androit Bone	Deep insert to 22.02	Perpendicular insertion. Nourishes Qi. **Do not use on pregnant patient.**
Quinsy	**77.24** **77.25**	**Zu Qian Jin** **Zu Wu Jin**	**Foot 1000 Gold** **Foot 5 Gold**	**0.5-1.0 cun** **0.5-1.0 cun**	**Perpendicular insertion.**
Regurgitation	77.09	Si Hua Zhong	4 Middle Flowers	Micro-puncture	See section on micro-puncture.
	77.17 77.18	Tian Huang Shen Guan	Heaven Emperor Kidney Gate	1.5-2 cun 0.5-1 cun	Perpendicular insertion. **Do not use 77.17 on pregnant patients.**
	1010.07	Zong Shu	Total Pivot	Micro-puncture	Insert downward. See section on micro-puncture.
Renal calculus with renal colic pain	22.07	Xia Bai	Lower White	0.3-0.5 cun	Perpendicular insertion.

Tung Acupuncture: A Quick Reference Guide

Indications	Point #	Name Pinyin	Name English	Insertion	Comments
Renal calculus Acute & chronic	1010.13	Ma Jin Shui	Horse Gold Water	0.1-0.3 cun	Perpendicular insertion. Add 1010.14 to enhance the therapeutic effect.
Renal colic	1010.13 22.07	Ma Jin Shui Xia Bai	Horse Gold Water Lower White	0.1-0.3 cun 0.3-0.5 cun	Perpendicular insertion. Needle 22.07 along bone. This combination is very effective.
Renal disorders	77.18 77.19 77.21	Shen Guan Di Huang Ren Huang	Kidney Gate Earthly Emperor Man Emperor	0.8-2.5 cun 1.0-1.5 cun 0.6-1.2 cun	Perpendicular insertion. **Do not use 77.19, 77.21 on pregnant patients.**
Renal inflammation	88.09 88.10 88.11	Tong Shen Tong Wei Tong Bei	Passing Kidney Passing Stomach Passing Back	0.3-0.5 cun 0.3-0.8 cun 0.5-1.0 cun	Perpendicular insertion. Pick 2 of these 3 points (4 points at 2 thighs), Never use 3 needles same time. Help prevent miscarriage.
Renal pain	**11.12**	**Er Jiao Ming**	**Two Corner Bright**	**0.1 cun**	**Use both points.**
Renal stones	**22.07**	**Xia Bai**	Lower White	**0.3-0.5 cun**	**Perpendicular insertion. (Cholic pain)**
	44.17	Shui Yu	Water Cure	Micro-puncture	See section on micro-puncture.
Restless	77.09	Si Hua Zhong	4 Middle Flowers	Micro-puncture	See section on micro-puncture.
Restriction of neck movement	**66.11**	**Huo Ju**	**Fire Chrysanthemum**	**0.5-0.8 cun**	**Horizontal insertion. Do not use on pregnant patient. Use on one side only.**
Retro version of uterus	11.06	Huan Chao	Return Nest	0.3 cun	Vertical insertion along bone. Either side, but not both.
Rheumatic fever (Esp. arthritis)	**88.01** **88.02** **88.03**	**Tong Guan** **Tong Shan** **Tong Tian**	**Penetrating Gate** **Passing Mountain** **Passing Sky**	**0.3-0.5 cun** **0.5-0.8 cun** **0.5-1.0 cun**	**Perpendicular insertion.**
Rheumatic heart disease	**11.19**	**Xin Chang**	**Heart Normal**	**0.1-0.2 cun**	**Perpendicular insertion, use both points.**
	11.16	Huo Xi	Fire Knee	0.1 cun	Micro-puncture along spinal column region.
Rheumatism	1010.23 1010.24	Zhou Huo Zhou Jin	Prefect Fire Prefect Gold	0.1-0.3 cun 0.1-0.3 cun	Perpendicular insertion.
Rheumatoid arthritis	11.22	Fu Yuan	Recover	0.1 cun	Perpendicular insertion. Use all 3 points. Effective for RA bone expansion.
	11.27	Wu Hu	Five Tigers	0.2 cun	Perpendicular insertion. Lower body pain, ie. Feet. Use up to 3 needles.

Notes:

69

Tung Acupuncture: A Quick Reference Guide

Indications	Point #	Name Pinyin	Name English	Insertion	Comments
Rhinitis	11.07	**Zhi Si Ma**	**Finger 4 Horse**	**0.1 cun**	**Perpendicular insertion. Use all 3 points.**
	44.01	**Fen Jin**	**Dividing Gold**	**0.5-1.0 cun**	**Perpendicular insertion.**
	88.17 88.18 88.19	**Zi Ma Zhong** **Zi Ma Shang** **Zi Ma Xia**	**Center 4 Horses** **Upper 4 Horses** **Lower 4 Horses**	**0.8-2.5 cun.** **0.8-2.5 cun** **0.8-2.5 cun**	**Perpendicular insertion. Can treat all types of nasal diseases. Mild cases need a few tx. Severe cases require more tx with longer retention.**
	11.17	**Mu**	**Wood**	**0.25 cun**	**Shallow insertion, but still touch periosteum. Pinch point before insertion b/c painful. (Acute)**
	33.07	Huo Fu Hai	Fire Bowels	0.5-1.0 cun	Perpendicular insertion. For systemic disease do bilaterally.
	33.15	Tian Shi	Heaven Scholar	1.0-1.5 cun	Perpendicular insertion.
	1010.13	Ma Jin Shui	Horse Gold Water	0.1-0.3 cun	Perpendicular insertion. Right side is more effective than left side. Use right side if patient is right handed.
	1010.14	Ma Kuai Shui	Horse Fast Water	0.1-0.3 cun	Perpendicular insertion.
	1010.12	Zheng Ben	Upright Source	0.1-0.2 cun	Perpendicular. (Allergic)
Rib pain	11.07 77.05 77.06 77.07 77.26	**Zhi Si Ma** **Yi Zhong** **Er Zhong** **San Zhong** **Qi Hu**	**Finger 4 Horse** **First Weight** **Second Weight** **Third Weight** **Seven Tigers**	**0.1 cun** **1.0-2.0 cun** **1.0-2.0 cun** **1.0-2.0 cun** **0.5-0.8 cun**	**Perpendicular insertion.**
Rib pain (costaglia)	VT03	King Wu	Gold Five	Micro-puncture	Mostly due to infection. See section on micro-puncture.
Scabies	DT01 DT02	Fen Chi Shang Fen Chi Sha	Upper Separation Branch Lower Separation Branch	1.0-1.5 cun 0.5-1.0 cun	Perpendicular insertion. Bilateral
Scanty menstruation	11.24	**Fu Ke**	**Lady Class**	**0.2 cun**	**Diagonal towards index finger.**
Scapulalgia	11.09	**Xin Xi**	**Heart Knee**	**0.1 cun**	**Perpendicular insertion. Use both points. Next to the bone.**
	77.26	**Qi Hu**	**Seven Tigers**	**0.5-0.8 cun**	**Perpendicular insertion. Use all 3 points at same time contra lateral. Similar to 5 tigers 11.27.**
Scapular muscle pain	22.01	Zhong Zi	Double Son	1.0-1.5cun	Perpendicular insertion.
Scapular pain	11.28	**Bei Tong**	**Back Pain**	**0.1 cun**	**Perpendicular.**
	11.09 11.28 22.01 77.26	**Xin Xi** **Bei Tong** **Zhong Zi** **Qi Hu**	**Heart Knee** **Back Pain** **Double Son** **Seven Tigers**	**0.1 cun** **0.1 cun** **1.0-1.5 cun** **0.5-0.8 cun**	**Perpendicular insertion. Use both points of 11.09 next to the bone. Use all 3 points of 77.26 at same time contra lateral.**
	77.14	**Si Hua Wai**	**4 Lateral Flowers**	**1.0-1.5 cun**	**Perpendicular insertion 28g or Micro-puncture**
	77.04	Bo Qiu	Catching Ball	1.0-2.0 cun	Image popleteal - scapula.

70

Indications	Point #	Name Pinyin	Name English	Insertion	Comments
Sciatica	22.04 22.05	Da Bai Ling Gu	Big White Androit Bone	Deep insert to 22.01 Deep insert to 22.02	**Perpendicular insertion.Special effect.** **If the pain is along the ST meridian, add 66.05. Do not use on pregnant patients.**
	33.05 1010.02 1010.03 1010.04	Huo Ling Zhou Yuan Zhou Kun Zhou Lun	Fire Mound Prefecture Round Prefecture Elder Brother Prefecture Mountain	0.5-1.0 cun 0.1-0.3 cun 0.1-0.3 cun 0.1-0.3 cun	**Perpendicular insertion.**
	33.04 33.05 33.06	Huo Chuan Huo Ling Huo Shan	Fire Threaded Fire Mound Fire Mountain	0.3-0.5 cun 0.5-1.0 cun 1.0-1.5 cun	**Perpendicular insertion.**
	55.04	Hua Gu San	Flower Bone 3	0.8 cun	**Perpendicular insertion.**
	88.17 88.18 88.19	Zi Ma Zhong Zi Ma Shang Zi Ma Xia	Center 4 Horses Upper 4 Horses Lower 4 Horses	0.8-2.5 cun. 0.8-2.5 cun 0.8-2.5 cun	**Perpendicular insertion.**
	99.05	Jin Er	Gold Ear	0.2 cun	**Top ¼ of lobe. Same mechanism as scoliosis.**
	1010.22	Bi Yi	Nasal Wing	0.1-0.2 cun	**Perpendicular insertion.**
	88.12 77.09 77.11	**Ming Huang** Si Hua Zhong Si Hua Xia	**Bright Yellow** 4 Middle Flowers 4 Lower Flowers	1.5-2.5 cun Micro-puncture 0.5-1.0 cun	**Perpendicular insertion.** See section on micro-puncture. **Needle along the bone. (Due to bone spurs)**
	22.03	Shang Bai	Upper White	0.3-0.5 cun	Perpendicular insertion. Bidirectional as needed. **Do not use on pregnant patients.**
	22.06	Zhong Bai	Center White	0.3-0.5 cun	Perpendicular insertion. Can also use 11.21, 1010.22
	22.07	Xia Bai	Lower White	0.3-0.5 cun	Perpendicular insertion.
	33.07 33.08	Huo Fu Hai Shou Wu Jin	Fire Bowels Hand Five Gold	0.5-1.0 cun 0.3-0.5 cun	Always use with 33.09. For systemic disease do bilaterally.
	33.08 33.09	Shou Wu Jin Shou Qian Jin	Hand Five Gold Hand 1000 Gold	0.3-0.5 cun 0.3-0.5 cun	Perpendicular insertion.
	44.15	Xia Qu	Lower Curve	0.6-1.0 cun	Perpendicular insertion.
	44.16	Shang Qu	Upper Curve	0.6-1.5 cun	Perpendicular insertion.
	55.05	Hua Gu Si	Flower Bone 4	0.5-1.0 cun	Perpendicular insertion.
	77.03	Zheng Shi	Upright Scholar	0.5-1.0 cun	Perpendicular insertion. Through the Achilles tendon.
	1010.21	Yu Huo	Jade Fire	0.1-0.3 cun	Perpendicular insertion.
	1010.24	Zhou Jin	Prefect Gold	0.1-0.3 cun	Perpendicular insertion.
	22.08 22.09	Wan Shun Yi Wan Shun Er	Wrist Flow One Wrist Flow Two	1.0-1.5 cun 1.0-1.5 cun	Perpendicular insertion. Esp. for female but only pick in one hand.
	DT09	Jin Lin	Gold Forest	Micro-puncture	See section on micro-puncture.

Tung Acupuncture: A Quick Reference Guide

Indications	Point #	Name Pinyin	Name English	Insertion	Comments
Sciatica Due to lung deficiency	22.04	Da Bai	Big White	Deep insert to 22.01	Perpendicular insertion. **Do not use on pregnant patient.**
	22.05	Ling Gu	Android Bone	Deep insert to 22.02	Perpendicular insertion. **Do not use on pregnant patient.**
	88.17 88.18 88.19	Zi Ma Zhong Zi Ma Shang Zi Ma Xia	Center 4 Horses Upper 4 Horses Lower 4 Horses	0.8-2.5 cun. 0.8-2.5 cun 0.8-2.5 cun	Perpendicular insertion. Contral ateral
Sciatica Along GB Meridian	77.14	Si Hua Wai	4 Lateral Flowers	Micro-puncture	Black blood to treat acute enteritis, intercostals neuralgia, chest oppression, asthma, sciatica (along GB meridian) and other neuralgia. See section on micro-puncture.
Scoliosis	**99.05**	**Jin Er**	**Gold Ear**	**0.2 cun**	**Top ¼ of lobe. Do not treat if angle is greater than 45º; send out, it is a surgical matter. Scoliosis (Esp. abnormal lumbar curve)**
	99.05 1010.06 1010.22	**Jin Er Hou Hui Bi Yi**	**Gold Ear Posterior Meetings Nasal Wing**	**0.2 cun 0.1-0.3 cun 0.1-0.2 cun**	**Perpendicular insertion. Add 44.06 and dao ma with points 2cun & 4 cun below 44.06 for a total of 3 extra points to enhance the therapeutic effect.**
	88.03 88.12 88.14	Tong Tian Ming Huang Qu Huang	Passing Sky Bright Yellow This Yellow	0.5-1.0 cun 1.5-2.5 cun 1.5-2.0 cun	Perpendicular insertion.
Seizure in children	**1010.01**	**Zheng Hui**	**Uprightness Meeting**	**0.1-0.3 cun**	**Horizontal insertion. Add 1010.08. Angle and direction of insertion is anterior to posterior insert 60º-90º.**
Seminal emissions	77.18 77.19 77.21	Shen Guan Di Huang Ren Huang	Kidney Gate Earthly Emperor Man Emperor	0.8-2.5 cun 1.0-1.5 cun 0.6-1.2 cun	Perpendicular insertion. **Do not use 77.19, 77.21 on pregnant patients.**
Sexual neurosis	**11.15**	**Zhi Shen**	**Finger Kidney**	**0.1 cun**	**Perpenducular insertion. Use all 3 points.**
Shen-K'uei syndrome	**77.18**	**Shen Guan**	**Kidney Gate**	**1.5-2 cun**	**Perpendicular insertion. Symptoms: Impotence, premature ejac., lack of concentration, decreased appetite, anemic in appearance, BPH**
	1010.19	Shui Tong	Water Through	0.1-0.5 cun	Horizontal insertion. Bilateral. Needle to the lateral side of chin. Add 77.18 to balance Kidney Y-Y.
	1010.20	Shiu Jin	Water Gold	0.1-0.5 cun	Horizontal insertion. Bilateral.
Shingles	**77.18 77.27**	**Shen Guan** Wai San Guan	**Kidney Gate Outer 3 Gates**	**0.8-2.5 cun 0.5-1.0 cun**	**Perpendicular insertion. Can Dao-Ma with 77.17. Do bilateral for a total of 8 needles.**

Notes:

Tung Acupuncture: A Quick Reference Guide

Indications	Point #	Name Pinyin	Name English	Insertion	Comments
Shock	**44.09**	**Di Zong**	**Earth Ancestor**	**1.0-2.0 cun**	**Perpendicular insertion. Recovering point. Always use both sides for better results. 1.0 cun insertion for minor issues, 2.0 cun insertion for critical conditions. (Most imporGall Bladdert point)**
	1010.05	Qian Hui	Anterior Meeting	0.1-0.3 cun	Anterior to posterior. (Esp. neurogenic type)
Shoulder & back pain	22.01	Zhong Zi	Double Son	1.0-1.5 cun	Perpendicular insertion.
	77.18	Shen Guan	Kidney Gate	0.8-2.5 cun	Perpendicular insertion.
	88.09	Tong Shen	Passing Kidney	0.3-0.5 cun	Perpendicular insertion.
	88.10	Tong Wei	Passing Stomach	0.3-0.8 cun	
	88.11	Tong Bei	Passing Back	0.5-1.0 cun	
Shoulder difficlty lifting	33.16	Qu Ling	Curved Mound	0.3-0.5 cun	Perpendicular insertion. Effective with reducing method manipulation.
	55.03	Hua Gu Er	Flower Bone 2	0.5-1.0 cun	Perpendicular insertion.
	77.08	Si Hua Shang	4 Upper Flowers	2.0-3.0 cun	Perpendicular insertion. Either side is effective, but mostly contralateral. Ipsilateral is effective. See section on micro-puncture.
	77.09	Si Hua Zhong	4 Middle Flowers	Micro-puncture	
	77.18	Shen Guan	Kidney Gate	0.8-2.5 cun	Perpendicular insertion. Contralateral has special effect. Can also Micro-puncture
	77.24	Zu Qian Jin	Foot 1000 Gold	0.5-1.0 cun	Perpendicular insertion. Has special effect, for difficulty touhing the scapula.
	77.25	Zu Wu Jin	Foot 5 Gold	0.5-1.0 cun	
Shoulder frozen	**33.13**	**Ren Shi**	**Human Scholar**	**0.5-1.0 cun**	**Perpendicular insertion.**
	77.09	**Si Hua Zhong**	**4 Middle Flowers**	**Micro-puncture**	**Perpendicular insertion contralateral. If still can't move, micro-pucture ipsilateral.**
	77.13	**Si Hua Li**	**4 Inner Flowers**	**1.5-2.0 cun**	
	77.14	**Si Hua Wai**	**4 Lateral Flowers**	**1.0-1.5 cun**	
	77.27	Wai San Guan	Outer 3 Gates	1.0-1.5 cun.	Perpendicular insertion. Similar to 5 tigers 11.27.
Shoulder joint pain	77.18	Shen Guan	Kidney Gate	0.8-2.5 cun	Perpendicular insertion. Add the corresponding shu-stream point for better results.
Shoulder joint sprain	44.06	Jian Zhong	Shoulder Center	1.0-1.5 cun	Perpendicular insertion.
Shoulder pain	**33.13**	**Ren Shi**	**Human Scholar**	**0.5-1.0 cun**	**Perpendicular insertion. (Any pain from shoulder to wrist & scapula)**
	77.27	**Wai San Guan**	**Outer 3 Gates**	**1.0-1.5 cun**	
	88.04	**Jie Mei Yi**	**First Sister**	**1.5-2.0 cun**	
	88.11	**Tong Bei**	**Passing Back**	**0.5-1.0 cun**	
	1010.21	**Yu Huo**	**Jade Fire**	**0.1-0.3 cun**	
	22.14	San Cha San	Three Jam Three	1.0 – 1.5 cun	Needle on diseased side. Towards the palm.
	44.06	Jian Zhong	Shoulder Center	1.0-1.5 cun	Perpendicular insertion.
	88.25	Zhong Jiu Li	Middle 9 Miles	0.8-2.0 cun	Perpendicular insertion.
	88.26	Shang Jiu Li	Upper 9 Miles	0.8-2.0 cun	
	88.27	Xia Jiu Li	Lower 9 Miles	0.8-2.0 cun	
	1010.21	Yu Huo	Jade Fire	0.1-0.3 cun	Perpendicular insertion. 0.5 cun lateral from nose.
	DT16	Huang Ho	Paired Rivers	Micro-puncture	See section on micro-puncture.

73

Indications	Point #	Name Pinyin	Name English	Insertion	Comments
Shoulder problems	44.06	Jian Zhong	Shoulder Center	1.0-1.5 cun	Perpendicular insertion. Contralateral side.
Shoulder-arm pain	11.27	Wu Hu	Five Tigers	0.2 cun	Perpendicular insertion. Use 3 points.
	77.14	Si Hua Wai	4 Lateral Flowers	1.0-1.5 cun	Perpendicular insertion.
Shoulder-hand pain	**44.06**	**Jian Zhong**	**Shoulder Center**	**1.0-1.5 cun**	**Perpendicular insertion. Contra lateral.** **Middle of deltoid muscle.**
	77.03	Zheng Shi	Upright Scholar	0.5-1.0 cun	Perpendicular insertion. Through the Achilles tendon.
	88.25	Zhong Jiu Li	Middle 9 Miles	0.8-2.0 cun	Perpendicular insertion. Right side is
	88.26	Shang Jiu Li	Upper 9 Miles	0.8-2.0 cun	more powerful than left side.
Sinus pain (At cartilage & bone)	**11.12**	**Er Jiao Ming**	**Two Corner Bright**	**0.1 cun**	**Towards the small finger is very effective. Use both points.**
Sinusitis	**88.17**	**Zi Ma Zhong**	**Center 4 Horses**	**0.8-2.5 cun.**	**Perpendicular insertion. Can treat**
	88.18	**Zi Ma Shang**	**Upper 4 Horses**	**0.8-2.5 cun**	**all types of nasal diseases. Mild**
	88.19	**Zi Ma Xia**	**Lower 4 Horses**	**0.8-2.5 cun**	**cases need a few tx. Severe cases require more tx with longer retention.**
Skin allergy	**88.23**	**Jin Qian Xia**	**Lower Gold Front**	**0.3-0.5 cun**	**Perpendicular insertion.**
	88.24	Jin Qian Shang	Upper Gold Front	0.5-1.0 cun	Perpendicular insertion.
Skin conditions	88.17	Zi Ma Zhong	Center 4 Horses	0.8-2.5 cun.	Perpendicular insertion.
	88.18	Zi Ma Shang	Upper 4 Horses	0.8-2.5 cun	
	88.19	Zi Ma Xia	Lower 4 Horses	0.8-2.5 cun	
Skin diseases	**44.05**	**Hou Zhi**	**Back Branch**	**0.3-0.7 cun**	**Perpendicular insertion. Add 11.07.** **(All major)**
	Ear	Apex		Micro-puncture	See section on micro-puncture.
	88.17	Zi Ma Zhong	Center 4 Horses	0.8-2.5 cun.	Perpendicular insertion.
	88.18	Zi Ma Shang	Upper 4 Horses	0.8-2.5 cun	
	88.19	Zi Ma Xia	Lower 4 Horses	0.8-2.5 cun	
Skin disorder (Esp. neck skin)	44.06	Jian Zhong	Shoulder Center	1.0-1.5 cun	Perpendicular insertion.
Skin infection (Erysipelas)	88.01	Tong Guan	Penetrating Gate	0.3-0.5 cun	Perpendicular insertion.
	88.02	Tong Shan	Passing Mountain	0.5-0.8 cun	
	88.03	Tong Tian	Passing Sky	0.5-1.0 cun	
Skin snsitiveness	Ear	Apex		Micro-puncture	See section on micro-puncture.
	88.17	Zi Ma Zhong	Center 4 Horses	0.8-2.5 cun.	Perpendicular insertion.
	88.18	Zi Ma Shang	Upper 4 Horses	0.8-2.5 cun	
	88.19	Zi Ma Xia	Lower 4 Horses	0.8-2.5 cun	
Slipped disc	**44.03**	**Shou Ying**	**Head Wisdom**	**0.3-0.5 cun**	**Perpendicular insertion. Use with 44.02.**
Smoking cessation	88.18	Zi Ma Shang	Upper 4 Horses	0.8-2.5 cun	Perpendicular insertion.
Sore throat	22.14	San Cha San	Three Jam Three	1.0 – 1.5 cun	Very effective 22.14 Towards the palm.
	22.11	Tu Shui	Earth Water	0.2-0.3 cun	22.11 perpendicular.
	77.24	Zu Qian Jin	Foot 1000 Gold	0.5-1.0 cun	Perpendicular insertion.
	77.25	Zu Wu Jin	Foot 5 Gold	0.5-1.0 cun	
	VT01	Huo O Chiu	Throat Moth 9	Micro-puncture	**Use extreme caution:** do not damage the cartilage or Thyroid gland. See section on micro-puncture.

Indications	Point #	Name Pinyin	Name English	Insertion	Comments
Soreness of the hand	77.22 77.23	Ce San Li Ce Xia San Li	Lateral 3 Mile Below Lateral 3 Mile	0.5-1.0 cun 0.5-1.0 cun	Perpendicular insertion. Ipsilateral treatment. Bilateral for sornes of both hands
Spasm of the hand tendon issue	22.01 22.02	Zhong Zi Zhong Xian	Double Son Double Saint	1.0-1.5 cun 1.0-1.5 cun	Perpendicular insertion. Add 77.18 to enhance the results.
	33.16	Qu Ling	Curved Mound	0.3-0.5 cun	Perpendicular insertion. Reducing method, then needle 77.18.
Speaking trouble	**1010.22**	**Bi Yi**	**Nasal Wing**	**0.1-0.2 cun**	**Perpendicular insertion.** **Vocal chord problems.**
Spinal pain	**44.02**	**Hou Zhui**	**Back Vertibrae**	**0.3-0.5 cun**	**Perpendicular insertion. Use with 44.03.**
	44.02 **44.03** **77.01** **77.02** **77.03**	**Hou Zhui** **Shou Ying** **Zheng Jin** **Zheng Zong** **Zheng Shi**	**Back Vertibrae** **Head Wisdom** **Upright Tendon** **Uprightness Ancestry** **Upright Scholar**	**0.3-0.5 cun** **0.3-0.5 cun** **0.5-0.8 cun** **0.5-0.8 cun** **0.5-1.0 cun**	**Perpendicular insertion.**
	55.04	**Hua Gu San**	**Flower Bone 3**	**0.8 cun**	**Perpendicular insertion.**
	66.14 **66.15**	**Shui Xiang** **Shui Xian**	**Water Phase** **Water Fairy**	**0. 3-.05 cun** **0.5 cun**	**Perpendicular insertion. Through anterior margin of the tendon. Insertion through flexor tetinaculum.**
	77.01 **77.02**	**Zheng Jin** **Zheng Zong**	**Upright Tendon** **Uprightness Ancestry**	**0.5-0.8 cun** **0.5-0.8 cun**	**Perpendicular insertion. Through the Achilles tendon. Add 22.08 accessory point for neck pain. Contra lateral insertion first, then ipsi lateral insertion. Always use 77.02 with 77.01 for better results. Add 22.08. (Neck)**
	22.05	Ling Gu	Android Bone	Deep insert to 22.02	Perpendicular insertion. Bidirectional as needed. **Do not use on pregnant patient.**
	55.05	Hua Gu Si	Flower Bone 4	0.5-1.0 cun	Perpendicular insertion.
	88.14 88.15 88.16	Qi Huang Huo Zhi Huo Quan	This Yellow Fire Branch Fire Complete	1.5-2.0 cun 1.5-2.0 cun 1.5-2.0 cun	Perpendicular insertion.
	88.16	Huo Quan	Fire Complete	1.5-2.0 cun	Perpendicular insertion.
	1010.06	Hou Hui	Posterior Meetings	0.1-0.3 cun	Insertion downward. (Esp. thoracic lumbar)
	1010.14	Ma Kuai Shui	Horse Fast Water	0.1-0.3 cun	Perpendicular insertion.
	1010.25	Zhou Shui	Prefect Water	0.1-0.3 cun	Insert upward or downward, use 2 needles.
	L1	Shui Chung	Water Center	0.8-1.0 cun	Perpendicular insertion.
	77.01 77.02	Zheng Jin Zheng Zong	Upright Tendon Uprightness Ancestry	0.5-0.8 cun 0.5-0.8 cun	Perpendicular insertion. Left for males, right for females. If no effect, do contralateral. (Pain along the midline)
Spinal sprain acute	22.08	Wan Sun Yi	Wrist Flow One	1.0-1.5 cun	Perpendicular.
	77.01 77.04	Zheng Jin Bo Qiu	Upright Tendon Catching Ball	0.5-0.8 cun 1.0-2.0 cun	Perpendicular insertion.

75

Tung Acupuncture: A Quick Reference Guide

Indications	Point #	Name Pinyin	Name English	Insertion	Comments
Spinal vertebra tenderness	77.09 77.10	Si Hua Zhong Si Hua Fu	4 Middle Flowers 4 Append Flowers	Micro-puncture Micro-puncture	See section on micro-puncture or needle. Needle along the bone.
	88.25 88.26 88.27	Zhong Jiu Li Shang Jiu Li Xia Jiu Li	Middle 9 Miles Upper 9 Miles Lower 9 Miles	0.8-2.0 cun 0.8-2.0 cun 0.8-2.0 cun	Perpendicular insertion. Add 22.08 to enhance the effect.
Spinal vertebrae spur	**88.12**	**Ming Huang**	**Bright Yellow**	**1.5-2.5 cun**	**Perpendicular insertion.**
	22.08	Wan Shun Yi	Wrist Flow One	1.0-1.5 cun	Perpendicular insertion. Tonify Kidney to TX spurs.
	77.09 77.10	Si Hua Zhong Si Hua Fu	4 Middle Flowers 4 Append Flowers	Micro-puncture Micro-puncture	See section on micro-puncture. Needle along the bone. Good for cervical & thoracic spurs.
	88.25	Zhong Jiu Li	Middle 9 Miles	0.8-2.0 cun	Perpendicular insertion.
	88.25 88.26 88.27	Zhong Jiu Li Shang Jiu Li Xia Jiu Li	Middle 9 Miles Upper 9 Miles Lower 9 Miles	0.8-2.0 cun 0.8-2.0 cun 0.8-2.0 cun	Perpendicular insertion. Add 22.08 to enhance the effect.
	22.08 88.25	Wan Shun Yi Zhong Jiu Li	Wrist Flow One Middle 9 Miles	1.0-1.5 cun 0.8-2.0 cun	Perpendicular.
Spleen disharmony	66.06 66.07	Mu Liu Mu Dou	Wood Stay Wood Scoop	0.3-0.5 cun 0.3-0.5 cun	Perpendicular insertion.
Spleen enlargement	44.08	Ren Zong	Man Ancestor	1.2 cun	Perpendicular insertion. Caution Biceps muscle or Cephalic vein.
Spleen strengthen supplement Qi	88.17 88.18 88.19	Zi Ma Zhong Zi Ma Shang Zi Ma Xia	Center 4 Horses Upper 4 Horses Lower 4 Horses	0.8-2.5 cun. 0.8-2.5 cun 0.8-2.5 cun	Perpendicular insertion.
Splenitis	11.18	Pi Zhong	Spleen Edema	0.1 cun	Perpendicular insertion.
Splenomegaly	**11.18**	**Pi Zhong**	**Spleen Edema**	**0.1 cun**	**Perpendicular insertion.**
	66.06 **66.07**	**Mu Liu** **Mu Dou**	**Wood Stay** **Wood Scoop**	**0.3-0.5 cun** **0.3-0.5 cun**	**Perpendicular insertion.**
	77.05 **77.06** **77.07**	**Yi Zhong** **Er Zhong** **San Zhong**	**First Weight** **Second Weight** **Third Weight**	**1.0-2.0 cun** **1.0-2.0 cun** **1.0-2.0 cun**	**Perpendicular insertion.** **Use the right side only.** **77.05 projection point of 11.14.**
	44.08	Ren Zong	Man Ancestor	1.2 cun	Perpendicular insertion. Caution Biceps muscle or Cephalic vein.
	66.06	Mu Liu	Wood Stay	0.3-0.5 cun	Perpendicular insertion.
	66.07	Mu Dou	Wood Scoop	0.5-1.0 cun	Perpendicular insertion.
	66.06 66.07	Mu Liu Mu Dou	Wood Stay Wood Scoop	0.3-0.5 cun 0.3-0.5 cun	Perpendicular insertion. Add 77.07 for enhanced effect.
	77.07	San Zhong	Third Weight	Micro-puncture	See section on micro-puncture. Only use right side.
Splenopathy	**11.18**	**Pi Zhong**	**Spleen Edema**	**0.1 cun**	**Perpendicular insertion.**
Spondylaglia	**11.11**	**Fei Xin**	**Lung Heart**	**0.1 cun**	**Perpendicular insertion. Use both points.**
Spondylitis	88.12 88.13 88.14	Ming Huang Tian Huang Qi Huang	Bright Yellow Heavenly Yellow This Yellow	1.5-2.5 cun 1.5-2.5 cun 1.5-2.0 cun	Perpendicular insertion.
Spondylosis cervical	88.25	Zhong Jiu Li	Middle 9 Miles	0.8-2.0 cun	Perpendicular insertion. Right side is more powerful than left side.
Sports injury	11.27	Wu Hu	Five Tigers	0.2 cun	Perpendicular insertion. Lower body pain, ie. Feet. Use up to 3 needles.

Tung Acupuncture: A Quick Reference Guide

Indications	Point #	Name Pinyin	Name English	Insertion	Comments
Sprain neck	22.01	Zhong Zi	Double Son	1.0-1.5 cun	Perpendicular insertion. May only need a single treatment.
	22.14	San Cha San	Three Jam Three	1.0 – 1.5 cun	Towards the palm.
Spur of the heel	77.09 77.11	Si Hua Zhong Si Hua Xia	4 Middle Flowers 4 Lower Flowers	Micro-puncture	See section on micro-puncture. Perpendicular insertion. Insert needle close to the Tibia. Add 33.12 to improve the therapeutic effect.
Spur of the knee	77.09 77.11	Si Hua Zhong Si Hua Xia	4 Middle Flowers 4 Lower Flowers	Micro-puncture	See section on micro-puncture. Perpendicular insertion. Insert needle close to the Tibia. Add 33.12 to improve the therapeutic effect.
Spur spinal vertebrae	88.25 88.26 88.27	Zhong Jiu Li Shang Jiu Li Xia Jiu Li	Middle 9 Miles Upper 9 Miles Lower 9 Miles	0.8-2.0 cun 0.8-2.0 cun 0.8-2.0 cun	Perpendicular insertion. Add 22.08 to enhance the effect.
Spurs	77.09 77.10	Si Hua Zhong Si Hua Fu	4 Middle Flowers 4 Append Flowers	Micro-puncture Micro-puncture	See section on micro-puncture. Needle along the bone.
Squint	77.18	Shen Guan	Kidney Gate	0.8-2.5 cun	Perpendicular insertion.
Sterility	**66.02**	**Mu Fu**	**Wood Wife**	**0.2-0.4 cun**	**Perpendicular insertion. Use 30g-32g needle. Touch periosteum.** (Partial obstruction of Fallopian tubes) (Decreased sperm motility)
Sternum pain	**77.26**	**Qi Hu**	**Seven Tigers**	**0.5-0.8 cun**	**Perpendicular insertion. Use all 3 points at same time contra lateral. Similar to 5 tigers 11.27.**
Stomach diseases	66.04	Huo Zhu	Fire Master	0.3-0.8 cun	Perpendicular insertion. No moxa. **Do not use on pregnant patient.**
	66.05	Men Jin	Door Gold	0.5 cun	Perpendicular insertion. For male patients use left side only, for female patiens use right side. Can also Micro-puncture
	77.08	Si Hua Shang	4 Upper Flowers	Micro-puncture	See section on micro-puncture.
	77.09 77.14	Si Hua Zhong Si Hua Wai	4 Middle Flowers 4 Lateral Flowers	Micro-puncture 1.0-1.5 cun	See section on micro-puncture. Perpendicular insertion. You can also Micro-puncture
	88.01 88.02	Tong Guan Tong Shan	Penetrating Gate Passing Mountain	0.3-0.5 cun 0.5-0.8 cun	Perpendicular insertion. Micro-puncture initially, then needle to enchance the therapeutic result.
	VT04	Wei Mao Chi	Stomach Hair 7	Micro-puncture	See section on micro-puncture.
Stomach distension	**88.01 88.02**	**Tong Guan Tong Shan**	**Penetrating Gate Passing Mountain**	**0.3-0.5 cun 0.5-0.8 cun**	**Perpendicular insertion. Micro-puncture 77.09 first then needle 88.01 & 88.02.**
	33.12	Xin Men	Heart Gate	1.0-1.5 cun	Perpendicular insertion. Insert next to the bone. **Always use left arm.**
	66.05	Men Jin	Door Gold	0.5 cun	Perpendicular insertion. For male patients use left side only, for female patiens use right side. Can also Micro-puncture
Stomach ulceration	77.09 77.14	Si Hua Zhong Si Hua Wai	4 Middle Flowers 4 Lateral Flowers	Micro-puncture 1.0-1.5 cun	See section on micro-puncture. Perpendicular insertion. You can also Micro-puncture .

Indications	Point #	Name Pinyin	Name English	Insertion	Comments
Stomachache	**77.11** **77.12**	**Si Hua Xia** **Fu Chang**	**4 Lower Flowers** **Bowels Intestine**	**0.5-1.0 cun** **0.5-1.0 cun**	**Perpendicular insertion.** **Use 30g-32g needle not thicker.**
	11.03 11.04	Fu Jian Wai Jian	Floating Distance External Distance	0.1-0.2 cun 0.1-0.2 cun	All points perpendicular. Apply to right side.
	22.11	Tu Shui	Earth Water	0.2-0.3 cun	Perpendicular insertion. (Acute)
	55.05	Hua Gu Si	Flower Bone 4	0.5-1.0 cun	Perpendicular insertion.
	77.08 77.09	Si Hua Shang Si Hua Zhong	4 Upper Flowers 4 Middle Flowers	2.0-3.0 cun Micro-puncture	Perpendicular insertion. Both points together enhance the effect. See section on micro-puncture. (Acute)
	77.09 77.10	Si Hua Zhong Si Hua Fu	4 Middle Flowers 4 Append Flowers	Micro-puncture Micro-puncture	Right side has stronger effect. See section on micro-puncture.
	88.01 88.02 88.03	Tong Guan Tong Shan Tong Tian	Penetrating Gate Passing Mountain Passing Sky	0.3-0.5 cun 0.5-0.8 cun 0.5-1.0 cun	Perpendicular insertion. Only pick one or two points on one leg per treatment.
	DT04	Wu Ling	5 Mountain Ranges	Micro-puncture	See section on micro-puncture. (Acute)
Stop smoking	88.18	Zi Ma Shang	Upper 4 Horses	0.8-2.5 cun	Perpendicular insertion.
Strabismus	**77.18**	**Shen Guan**	**Kidney Gate**	**0.8-2.5 cun**	**Perpendicular insertion.** **Earlier treatment the better.**
	88.12	Ming Huang	Bright Yellow	1.5-2.5 cun	Perpendicular insertion. Micro-punture Taiyang increases recovery time. Do this every two weeks for up to 3 treatments.
Strangury	88.09 88.10 88.11	Tong Shen Tong Wei Tong Bei	Passing Kidney Passing Stomach Passing Back	0.3-0.5 cun 0.3-0.8 cun 0.5-1.0 cun	Perpendicular insertion. Pick 2 of these 3 points (4 points at 2 thighs), Never use 3 needles same time. Help prevent miscarriage.
Stress	**1010.01**	**Zheng Hui**	**Uprightness Meeting**	**0.1-0.3 cun**	**Horizontal insertion. Add 1010.08.** **Angle and direction of insertion is anterior to posterior insert 60°-90°.**
Stroke	**1010.01**	**Zheng Hui**	**Uprightness Meeting**	**0.1-0.3 cun**	**Horizontal insertion. Add 1010.08.** **Angle and direction of insertion is anterior to posterior insert 60°-90°.**
	DT04	Wu Ling	5 Mountain Ranges	Micro-puncture	See section on micro-puncture.
	1010.07	Zong Shu	Total Pivot	Micro-punture	Insert downward. (With aphasia)
	22.01 22.02	Zhong Zi Zhong Xian	Double Son Double Saint	1.0-1.5 cun 1.0-1.5 cun	Perpendicular insertion. Contralateral needling. (With hand convulsions)
	33.16	Qu Ling	Curved Mound	Micro-puncture	See section on micro-puncture. (With hand convulsions)
Stye	Ear	Apex		Micro-puncture	See section on micro-puncture.
	22.05	Ling Gu	Android Bone	Deep insert to 22.02	Perpendicular insertion. Contra lateral needling. 1-2 Tx can cure. **Do not use on pregnant patient.**
Sublingual swelling	Ear	Apex		Micro-puncture	See section on micro-puncture.
	77.22 77.23	Ce San Li Ce Xia San Li	Lateral 3 Mile Below Lateral 3 Mile	0.5-1.0 cun 0.5-1.0 cun	Perpendicular insertion. Bleeding jinjin & yuye extra may have even better result.
Sulaxation of joint (Due to falls and accident)	**44.15**	**Xia Qu**	**Lower Curve**	**0.6-1.0 cun**	**Perpendicular insertion.** **Add 77.26 (trauma point).**

Tung Acupuncture: A Quick Reference Guide

Indications	Point #	Name Pinyin	Name English	Insertion	Comments
Supra orbital pain	**1010.22**	**Bi Yi**	**Nasal Wing**	**0.1-0.2 cun**	**Perpendicular insertion.**
	11.12	**Er Jiao Ming**	**Two Corner Bright**	**0.1 cun**	**Use both points.**
Supraspinatus tendonitis	77.24	Zu Qian Jin	Foot 1000 Gold	0.5-1.0 cun.	Perpendicular insertion.
	77.25	Zu Wu Jin	Foot 5 Gold	0.5-1.0 cun	
Sweating excessive	**11.17**	**Mu**	**Wood**	**0.25 cun**	**Shallow insertion, but still touch periosteum. Pinch point before insertion b/c painful. Palm & feet. Can also be used for arm pit sweating.**
Swelling of legs	DT08	Jing Zhi	Essence Branch	Micro-puncture	See section on micro-puncture.
Syncope, iatrogenic	22.10	Shou Jie	Hand Release	0.5 cun	Perpendicular insertion. 0.5 cun insertion for 10 minutes. Micro-punture if you are in a hurry a couple drops of blood.
	88.28	**Jie**	**Release Point**	**0.3-0.5 cun**	**Perpendicular insertion. Not to exceed 5min. More powerful than 22.10**
Tachycardia	Ear	Apex		Micro-puncture	See section on micro-puncture.
	11.19	Xin Chang	Heart Normal	0.1-0.2 cun	Perpendicular insertion on 11.19, use both points. Perpendicular insertion on 33.12, close to bone only on left side. Add 22.14 to enhance the therapeutic effect.
	33.12	Xin Men	Heart Gate		
	22.14	San Cha San	Three Jam Three	1.0 – 1.5 cun	
	77.09	Si Hua Zhong	4 Middle Flowers	Micro-puncture	You can also Micro-puncture.
	77.14	Si Hua Wai	4 Lateral Flowers	1.0-1.5 cun	See section on micro-puncture.
Tarsal tunnel	**33.08**	**Shou Wu Jin**	Hand Five Gold	**0.3-0.5 cun**	**Perpendicular insertion.**
	33.09	**Shou Qian Jin**	Hand Thousand Gold	**0.3-0.5 cun**	
Teburculosis	77.09	Si Hua Zhong	4 Middle Flowers	Micro-puncture	Micro-puncture 77.09 & then needle 88.17, 88.18 & 88.19. Perpendicular insertion. See section on micro-puncture.
	77.14	Si Hua Wai	4 Lateral Flowers	Micro-puncture	
	88.17	Zi Ma Zhong	Center 4 Horses	0.8-2.5 cun	
	88.18	Zi Ma Shang	Upper 4 Horses	0.8-2.5 cun	
	88.19	Zi Ma Xia	Lower 4 Horses	0.8-2.5 cun	
Teeth clenching at night Bruxism	**77.11**	**Si Hua Xia**	**4 Lower Flowers**	**0.5-1.0 cun**	**Perpendicular insertion.**
	77.12	**Fu Chang**	**Bowels Intestine**	**0.5-1.0 cun**	**Use 30g-32g needle not thicker.**
Tendon diseases	22.05	Ling Gu	Androit Bone	Deep insert to 22.02	Perpendicular insertion. Insert needle along the bones. **Do not use these points on pregnant patient.**
	66.04	Huo Zhu	Fire Master	0.3-0.8 cun	
Tennis Elbow	**77.14**	**Si Hua Wai**	**4 Lateral Flowers**	**1.0-1.5 cun**	**Perpendicular insertion 28g or Micro-puncture**
	77.14	**Si Hua Wai**	**4 Lateral Flowers**	**1.0-1.5 cun**	**Perpendicular insertion.**
	77.18	**Shen Guan**	**Kidney Gate**	**1.5-2.0 cun**	
	DT16	Huang Ho	Paired Rivers	Micro-puncture	See section on micro-puncture.
Tenosynovitis	11.27	Wu Hu	Five Tigers	0.2 cun	Perpendicular insertion.
	77.22	Ce San Li	Lateral 3 Mile	0.5-1.0 cun	Perpendicular insertion.
Testitis	11.01	Da Jian	Big Distance	0.2-0.3 cun	All points perpendicular. Pick 2-3 points. Apply to right side.
	11.02	Xiao Jian	Small Distance	0.2-0.3 cun	
	11.03	Fu Jian	Floating Distance	0.1-0.2 cun	
	11.05	Zhong Jian	Center Distance	0.2-0.3 cun	

79

Indications	Point #	Name Pinyin	Name English	Insertion	Comments
Thigh pain	**88.25** **99.03**	**Zhong Jiu Li** **Huo Er**	**Middle 9 Miles** **Fire Ear**	**0.8-2.0 cun** **0.2 cun**	**Perpendicular insertion.**
	22.14	San Cha San	Three Jam Three	1.0 – 1.5 cun	Especially due to fatigue & over use. Ipsilateral towards the palm.
	22.14 88.26	San Cha San Shang Jiu Li	Three Jam Three Upper 9 Miles	1.0 – 1.5 cun 0.8-2.0 cun	22.14 towards the palm. 88.26 perpendicular.
	88.25 88.26 88.27	Zhong Jiu Li Shang Jiu Li Xia Jiu Li	Middle 9 Miles Upper 9 Miles Lower 9 Miles	0.8-2.0 cun 0.8-2.0 cun 0.8-2.0 cun	Perpendicular insertion.
	DT09	Jin Lin	Gold Forest	Micro-puncture	See section on micro-puncture.
Thigh pain and soreness	22.14	San Cha San	Three Jam Three	1.0 – 1.5 cun	May obtain best results. Towards the palm.
	44.06	Jian Zhong	Shoulder Center	1.0-1.5 cun	Perpendicular insertion.
	44.07	Bei Mian	Back Face	Micro-puncture	See section on micro-puncture.
	88.25 88.26 88.27	Zhong Jiu Li Shang Jiu Li Xia Jiu Li	Middle 9 Miles Upper 9 Miles Lower 9 Miles	0.8-2.0 cun 0.8-2.0 cun 0.8-2.0 cun	Contra lateral
	1010.19 1010.20	Shui Tong Shui Jin	Water Through Water Gold	0.1-0.5 cun 0.1-0.5 cun	Horizontal insertion. Bilateral.
	DT09	Jin Lin	Gold Forest	Micro-puncture	See section on micro-puncture.
Thirst	11.15	Zhi Shen	Finger Kidney	0.1 cun	Perpenducular insertion. Use all 3 points.
	L1 L2	Shui Chung Shui Fu	Water Center Water Bowels	0.8-1.0 cun 0.8-1.0 cun	Perpendicular insertion.
Throat itching	VT01	Huo O Chiu	Throat Moth 9	Micro-puncture	**Use extreme caution:** do not damage the cartilage or Thyroid gland. See section on micro-puncture.
Throat Sore	22.11 22.14	Tu Shui San Cha San	Earth Water Three Jam Three	0.2-0.3 cun 1.0 – 1.5 cun	Very effective 22.11 perpendicular. 22.14 Towards the palm.
Thrombocytopenia	55.05	Hua Gu Si	Flower Bone 4	0.5-1.0 cun	Perpendicular insertion.
Thumb pain (De Quervain's Tendonitis)	**66.01**	**Hai Bao**	**Seal**	**0.1-0.3 cun**	**Insert 66.01 perpendicularly and contralateral.**
Thyroid tumor	**88.32**	**Shi Yin**	**Voice Loss**	**1.0-1.5 cun**	**Horizontal insertion. Bilateral. Keep knee at 90° angle and have patient swallow for induction.**
Thyroiditis	**77.24** **77.25**	**Zu Qian Jin** **Zu Wu Jin**	**Foot 1000 Gold** **Foot 5 Gold**	**0.5-1.0 cun** **0.5-1.0 cun**	**Perpendicular insertion. Both points bilaterally. Add 77.24.**
	88.32	**Shi Yin**	**Voice Loss**	**1.0-1.5 cun**	**Horizontal insertion. Bilateral. Keep knee at 90° angle and have patient swallow for induction.**
	VT01	Huo O Chiu	Throat Moth 9	Micro-puncture	**Use extreme caution:** do not damage the cartilage or Thyroid gland. See section on micro-puncture.

Indications	Point #	Name Pinyin	Name English	Insertion	Comments
TIA	**88.29** **88.30** **88.31**	**Nei Tong Guan** **Nei Tong Shan** **Nei Tong Tian**	**Inner Passing Gate** **Inner Passing Mountain** **Inner Passing Sky**	**1.0 cun** **1.0 cun** **1.0 cun**	**Perpendicular insertion.**
	88.01 88.02 88.03	Tong Guan Tong Shan Tong Tian	Penetrating Gate Passing Mountain Passing Sky	0.3-0.5 cun 0.5-0.8 cun 0.5-1.0 cun	Perpendicular insertion.
Tic douroureaux	88.25	Zhong Jiu Li	Middle 9 Miles	0.8-2.0 cun	Perpendicular insertion. Right side is more powerful than left side.
Tics	**1010.01**	**Zheng Hui**	**Uprightness Meeting**	**0.1-0.3 cun**	**Horizontal insertion. Add 1010.08. Angle and direction of insertion is anterior to posterior insert 60°-90°.**
Tinea	11.17	Mu	Wood	0.25 cun	Shallow insertion, but still touch periosteum. Pinch point before insertion b/c painful.
Tinnitus	**11.07**	**Zhi Si Ma**	**Finger 4 Horse**	**0.1 cun**	**Perpendicular insertion. Use all 3 points.**
	55.02	**Hua Gu Yi**	**Flower Bone 1**	**0.5-1.0 cun**	**Perpendicular insertion, 30g or 32g needle. Equivalent to 22.05.**
	88.17 **88.18** **88.19**	**Zi Ma Zhong** **Zi Ma Shang** **Zi Ma Xia**	**Center 4 Horses** **Upper 4 Horses** **Lower 4 Horses**	**0.8-2.5 cun.** **0.8-2.5 cun** **0.8-2.5 cun**	**Perpendicular insertion. Best point 88.17.** **Needle Zi Ma with reducing method and needle Shen Guan with tonifying method.** **Combine with 22.05.**
	88.25	**Zhong Jiu Li**	**Middle 9 Miles**	**0.8-2.0 cun**	**Perpendicular insertion. Right side is more powerful than left side.**
	22.14	San Cha San	Three Jam Three	1.0 – 1.5 cun	Effective. Towards the palm.
	22.05	Ling Gu	Androit Bone	Deep insert to 22.02	Perpendicular insertion. Bidirectional as needed. Alternate with Zi Ma (**88.17, 88.18, 88.19**) **Do not use on pregnant patient.**
	22.08 22.09	Wa Shung Yi Wan Shun Er	Wrist Flow One Wrist Flow Two	1.0-1.5 cun 1.0-1.5 cun	Perpendicular insertion.
	33.16 88.12	Qu Ling Ming Huang	Curved Mound Bright Yellow	0.3-0.5 cun 1.5-2.5 cun	Perpendicular insertion. Needle 33.16 with reducing method and needle 88.12 with tonifying method.
Tiredness	**22.08** **22.09**	**Wan Shun Yi** **Wan Shun Er**	**Wrist Flow One** **Wrist Flow Two**	**1.0-1.5 cun** **1.0-1.5 cun**	**Perpendicular insertion.**
	44.07	**Bei Mian**	**Back Face**	**Micro-puncture**	**See section on micro-puncture.**
	1010.23	Zhou Huo	Prefect Fire	0.1-0.3 cun	Perpendicular insertion.
TMJ pain	**77.09**	**Si Hua Zhong**	4 Middle Flowers	**2.0-3.0 cun**	**Perpendicular insertion. You can also micropuncture this point.**
	66.03	Huo Ying	Fire Hardness	0.3-0.5 cun	Perpendicular insertion. **Do not use on pregnant patient.**
Toe numbness	11.27	Wu Hu	Five Tigers	0.2 cun	Perpendicular insertion. Needle the 3rd point.
	77.18 77.19 77.21	Shen Guan Di Huang Ren Huang	Kidney Gate Earthly Emperor Man Emperor	0.8-2.5 cun 1.0-1.5 cun 0.6-1.2 cun	Perpendicular insertion.. Needle 77.19 & 77.20, and then needle 77.18. **Do not use 77.19, 77.21 on pregnant patients.**
	DT05	Shuang Feng	Double Phoenix	Micro-puncture	See section on micro-puncture.

81

Tung Acupuncture: A Quick Reference Guide

Indications	Point #	Name Pinyin	Name English	Insertion	Comments
Toe pain	11.27	Wu Hu	Five Tigers	0.2 cun	Perpendicular insertion. Contra lateral
Toe pain due to gout	11.27	Wu Hu	Five Tigers	0.2 cun	Perpendicular insertion.
Tongue pain (heat related)	**1010.22**	**Bi Yi**	**Nasal Wing**	**0.1-0.2 cun**	**Perpendicular insertion.**
Tongue rigidity (Aphasia due to apoplexy)	44.06	Jian Zhong	Shoulder Center	1.0-1.5 cun	Perpendicular insertion.
	1010.07	Zong Shu	Total Pivot	0.1-0.2 cun	Insert downward. Needle shallow or Micro-puncture
	1010.19 1010.20	Shui Tong Shui Jin	Water Through Water Gold	0.1-0.5 cun 0.1-0.5 cun	Horizontal insertion. Bilateral.
Tonsillitis	**77.27**	Wai San Guan	**Outer 3 Gates**	**1.0-1.5 cun.**	**Perpendicular insertion. Similar to 5 tigers 11.27.**
	88.32	**Shi Yin**	**Voice Loss**	**1.0-1.5 cun**	**Horizontal insertion. Bilateral. Keep knee at 90° angle and have patient swallow for induction.**
	77.05 77.06 77.07	Yi Zhong Er Zhong San Zhong	First Weight Second Weight Third Weight	1.0-2.0 cun 1.0-2.0 cun 1.0-2.0 cun	Perpendicular insertion. Use all points bilaterally. 77.05 projection point of 11.14.
	77.24 77.25	Zu Qian Jin Zu Wu Jin	Foot 1000 Gold Foot 5 Gold	0.5-1.0 cun 0.5-1.0 cun	Perpendicular insertion.
Toothache	**77.14**	**Si Hua Wai**	**4 Lateral Flowers**	**1.0-1.5 cun**	**Perpendicular insertion 28g or Micro-puncture**
	77.22 **77.23**	**Ce San Li** **Ce Xia San Li**	**Lateral 3 Mile** **Below Lateral 3 Mile**	**0.5-1.0 cun** **0.5-1.0 cun**	**Perpendicular insertion.**
	11.03 11.04	Fu Jian Wai Jian	Floating Distance External Distance	0.1-0.2 cun 0.1-0.2 cun	All points perendicular. Apply to right side.
	22.05 77.22 77.23	Ling Gu Ce San Li Ce Xia San Li	Androit Bone Lateral 3 Mile Below Lateral 3 Mile	Deep insert to 22.02	Perpendicular insertion. 22.05 Bilaterally. 77.22 & 77.23 contra lateral **Do not use 22.05 on pregnant patient.**
	22.14	San Cha San	Three Jam Three	1.0 – 1.5 cun	Towards the palm.
	55.02	Hua Gu Yi	Flower Bone 1	0.5-1.0 cun	Perpendicular insertion, 30g or 32g needle. Equivalent to 22.05. (Upper & lower)
	77.08	Si Hua Shang	4 Upper Flowers	3.0-3.5 cun	Perpendicular insertion.
Tracheal obstruction	VT01	Huo O Chiu	Throat Moth 9	Micro-puncture	Due to sputum. **Use extreme caution:** do not damage the cartilage or Thyroid gland. See section on micro-puncture.
Trachoma (Eye infection)	55.02	Hua Gu Yi	Flower Bone 1	0.5-1.0 cun	Perpendicular insertion, 30g or 32g needle. Equivalent to 22.05.
Traumatic injury pain	**77.26**	**Qi Hu**	**Seven Tigers**	**0.5-0.8 cun**	**Perpendicular insertion. Use all 3 points at same time contra lateral. Similar to 5 tigers 11.27.**
	88.28	**Jie**	**Release Point**	**0.3-0.5 cun**	**Perpendicular insertion. (MVA, physical damage)**
Tremor (Due to anxiety, endocrine & MS)	**1010.08**	**Zhen Jing**	**Tranquility**	**0.1-0.2 cun**	**Located just above YinGall Bladderg, insert towards nose. Always use with 1010.01.**

82

Tung Acupuncture: A Quick Reference Guide

Indications	Point #	Name Pinyin	Name English	Insertion	Comments
Trigeminal neuralgia (Tic douloureaux)	55.06	Shang Liu	Upper Tumor	0.3-0.5 cun	Perpendicular insertion. Do not make deep insertion = dyspnea & discomfort.
	88.25	Zhong Jiu Li	Middle 9 Miles	0.8-2.0 cun	Perpendicular insertion. The right side is more powerful than left side.
Twitching of the eye	22.08 22.09	Wa Shun Yi Wan Shun Er	Wrist Flow One Wrist Flow Two	1.0-1.5 cun 1.0-1.5 cun	Perpendicular insertion.
	77.18 77.22 77.23	Shen Guan Ce San Li Ce Xia San Li	Kidney Gate Lateral 3 Mile Below Lateral 3 Mile	0.8-2.5 cun 0.5-1.0 cun 0.5-1.0 cun	Perpendicular insertion.
	88.20 88.21 88.22	Xia Quan Zhong Quan Shang Quan	Lower Fountain Middle Fountain Upper Fountain	0.3-0.5 cun 1.0-1.5 cun 1.0-1.5 cun	Perpendicular insertion.
Typhoid fever	VT02	Shi Er Hou	12 Monkeyes	Micro-puncture	Intestinal infection. See section on micro-puncture.
Ulcertation of the Duodenum	**77.09** 77.14	**Si Hua Zhong** **Si Hua Wai**	**4 Middle Flowers** **4 Lateral Flowers**	**Micro-puncture** **Micro-puncture**	**Also Micro-puncture visible veins on the dorsum of the foot. See section on micro-puncture.**
Ulnar neuritis (Numbness & tingling)	77.21	Ren Huang	Man Emperor	0.6-1.2 cun	Perpendicular insertion. **Do not use on pregnant patient.**
Umbilical pain	22.06 22.07	Zhong Bai Xia Bai	Center White Lower White	0.3-0.5 cun 0.3-0.5 cun	Perpendicular insertion.
	22.08 22.09	Wan Shun Yi Wan Shun Er	Wrist Flow One Wrist Flow Two	1.0-1.5 cun 1.0-1.5 cun	Perpendicular insertion. You can also use 22.06 & 22.07.
Ureterolith (Uriter stone)	**1010.16** **1010.17**	**Liu Kuai** **Qi Kuai**	**Six Fastness** **Seven Fastness**	**0.1-0.2 cun** **0.5-1.5 cun**	**Perpendicular insertion. Always use with 1010.14.**
Urethritis	11.03 11.04	Fu Jian Wai Jian	Floating Distance External Distance	0.1-0.2 cun 0.1-0.2 cun	All points perpendicular. Apply to right side.
	1010.16	Liu Kuai	Six Fastness	0.1-0.2 cun	Perpendicular insertion.
Urinary stones	**1010.14**	**Ma Kuai Shui**	**Horse Fast Water**	**0.1-0.3 cun**	**Perpendicular insertion. Fine stones can pass into bladder and get flush in urine.**
	66.03 66.04	Huo Ying Huo Zhu	Fire Hardness Fire Master	0.3-0.5 cun 0.3-0.8 cun	Perpendicular insertion. All good points for treatment. **Do not use on pregnant patients.**
Urination difficulty	**1010.14** **77.18**	**Ma Kuai Shu** **Shen Guan**	**Horse Fast Water** **Kidney Gate**	**0.1-0.3 cun** **1.5-2.0 cun**	**Perpendicular insertion. Pucture 1010.14 first then 77.18**
Urination frequent	**77.18**	**Shen Guan**	**Kidney Gate**	**0.8-2.5 cun**	**Perpendicular insertion.**
	66.01 66.02	Hai Bao Mu Fu	Seal Wood Wife	0.1-0.3 cun 0.2-0.4 cun	Perpendicular insertion.
	1010.14	Ma Kuai Shu	Horse Fast Water	0.1-0.3 cun	Perpendicular insertion.
Urithral calculus	1010.16 1010.17	Liu Kuai Qi Kuai	Six Fastness Seven Fastness	0.1-0.2 cun 0.5-1.5 cun	Perpendicular insertion.

Tung Acupuncture: A Quick Reference Guide

Indications	Point #	Name Pinyin	Name English	Insertion	Comments
Urticaria	99.07	Er Bei	Ear Back	Micro-puncture	See section on micro-puncture. Then needle 88.17-88.19 and 88.25-88.27.
	77.17	Tian Huang	Heaven Emperor	Micro-puncture	See section on micro-puncture. Micro-puncture between 77.17 & 77.21 and at 66.05. Then perpendicular.needle 88.17-88.19 and 88.25-88.27. You can also Micro-punture the back of the ear. For 66.05: For male patients use left side only, for female patiens use right side. Can also Micro-puncture **Do not use 77.17, 77.21 on pregnant patients.**
	77.21	Ren Huang	Man Emperor	Micro-puncture	
	66.05	Men Jin	Door Gold	0.5 cun	
	88.17	Zi Ma Zhong	Center 4 Horses	0.8-2.5 cun	
	88.18	Zi Ma Shang	Upper 4 Horses	0.8-2.5 cun	
	88.19	Zi Ma Xia	Lower 4 Horses	0.8-2.5 cun	
	88.25	Zhong Jiu Li	Upper 9 Miles	0.8-2.5 cun	
	88.26	Shang Jiu Li	Lower 9 Miles	0.8-2.5 cun	
	88.27	Xia Jiu Li		0.8-2.5 cun	
Urticaria on lower part of the body	88.25	Zhong Jiu Li	Middle 9 Miles	0.8-2.0 cun	Perpendicular insertion.
	88.26	Shang Jiu Li	Upper 9 Miles	0.8-2.0 cun	
	88.27	Xia Jiu Li	Lower 9 Miles	0.8-2.0 cun	
Urticaria on upper part of the body	44.06	Jian Zhong	Shoulder Center	1.0-1.5 cun	Perpendicular insertion.
Uterine inflammation (Metritis)	66.02	Mu Fu	Wood Wife	0.2-0.4 cun	Perpendicular insertion. Use 30g-32g needle. Touch periosteum.
	88.04	Jie Mei Yi	First Sister	1.5-2.0 cun	Perpendicular insertion.
Uterine myoma (Fibroids)	**11.06**	**Huan Chao**	**Return Nest**	**0.3 cun**	**Vertical insertion along bone. Either side, but not both.**
	66.13	**Shui Jing**	**Water Crystal**	**0.5-1.0 cun**	**Perpendicular insertion. Unilateral or bilateral through flexor retinaculum.**
	77.19	Di Huang	Earthly Emperor	1.0-1.5 cun	Perpendicular insertion. **Do not use on pregnant patient.**
Uterine pain	11.06	Huan Chao	Return Nest	0.3 cun	Vertical insertion along bone. Either side, but not both.
	88.09	Tong Shen	Passing Kidney	0.3-0.5 cun	Perpendicular insertion. Pick 2 of these 3 points (4 points at 2 thighs), Never use 3 needles same time. Help prevent miscarriage.
	88.10	Tong Wei	Passing Stomach	0.3-0.8 cun	
	88.11	Tong Bei	Passing Back	0.5-1.0 cun	
Uterine tumor	11.06	Huan Chao	Return Nest	0.3 cun	Vertical insertion along bone. Either side, but not both.
	11.24	Fu Ke	Lady Class	0.2 cun	Diagonal towards index finger.
	66.03	Huoying	Fire Hardness	0.3-0.5 cun	Perpendicular insertion. **Do not use on pregnant patients.**
	66.04	Huo Zhu	Fire Master	0.3-0.8 cun	Perpendicular insertion. No moxa. **Do not use on pregnant patients.**
Uterismus (Uterus pain)	11.24	Fu Ke	Lady Class	0.2 cun	Diagonal towards index finger.
Uteritis	11.06	Huan Chao	Return Nest	0.3 cun	Vertical insertion along bone. Either side, but not both.
	11.24	Fu Ke	Lady Class	0.2 cun	Diagonal towards index finger.
	DT15	San Chiang	Three Rivers	Micro-puncture	See section on micro-puncture.
	VT05	Fu Chao 23	Bowel Nest 23	Micro-puncture	See section on micro-puncture.
Uvulitis	**11.06**	**Huan Chao**	**Return Nest**	**0.3 cun**	**Vertical insertion along bone. Either side, but not both.**

84

Tung Acupuncture: A Quick Reference Guide

Indications	Point #	Name Pinyin	Name English	Insertion	Comments
Vaginal swelling	11.06	Huan Chao	Return Nest	0.3 cun	Vertical insertion along bone. Either side, but not both.
Vaginitis	**88.04** **88.05**	**Jie Mei Yi** **Jie Mei Er**	**First Sister** **Second Sister**	**1.5-2.0 cun** **1.5-2.5 cun**	**Perpendicular insertion.**
	11.24	Fu Ke	Lady Class	0.2 cun	Diagonal towards index finger.
	44.10	Tian Zong	Heaven Ancestor	1.0-1.5 cun	Perpendicular insertion. Caution Biceps muscle or Cephalic vein.
	44.11	Yun Bai	Cloud White	0.3-0.5 cun	Perpendicular insertion.
	44.11 66.01	Yun Bai Hai Bao	Cloud White Seal	0.3-0.5 cun 0.1-0.3 cun	Perpendicular insertion.
	66.01	Hai Bao	Seal	0.1-0.3 cun	Perpendicular insertion. Contra lateral.
	66.03 66.04	Huo Ying Huo Zhu	Fire Hardness Fire Master	0.3-0.5 cun 0.3-0.8 cun	Perpendicular insertion. **Do not use on pregnant patients.**
Vertigo	**22.05**	**Ling Gu**	**Androit Bone**	**Deep insert to 22.02**	**Perpendicular insertion. This is a very effective point. Do not use on pregnant patient.**
	77.18	**Shen Guan**	**Kidney Gate**	**0.8-2.5 cun**	**Perpendicular insertion.**
	66.10	Huo Lian	Fire Connection	0.5-0.8 cun	Horizontal insertion. **Do not use on pregnant patient.**
	66.11	Hou Ju	Fire Chrysanthemum	0.5-0.8 cun	Horizontal insertion. **Do not use on pregnant patient.**
	1010.19 1010.20	Shui Tong Shiu Jin	Water Through Water Gold	0.1-0.5 cun 0.1-0.5 cun	Horizontal insertion. Bilateral. Needle to the lateral side of chin. Add 77.18 to balance Kidney Y-Y. Bilaterally.
	1010.22	Bi Yi	Nasal Wing	0.1-0.2 cun	Perpendicular insertion.
	88.01 88.02	Tong Guan Tong Shan	Penetrating Gate Passing Mountain	0.3-0.5 cun 0.5-0.8 cun	Perpendicular insertion. (Due to anemia)
	77.18 77.19 77.21	Shen Guan Di Huang Ren Huang	Kidney Gate Earthly Emperor Man Emperor	0.8-2.5 cun 1.0-1.5 cun 0.6-1.2 cun	Perpendicular insertion. (Due to pathological changes of cerebral nerves). This combination supplements the Kidney **Do not use 77.19, 77.21 on pregnant patients.**
	22.05 77.07	Ling Gu San Zhong	Androit Bone Third Weight	Deep insert to 22.02 1.0-2.0 cun	Perpendicular insertion. Micro-puncture Improves cerebro-vascular circulation. (Severe case) **Do not use 22.05 on pregnant patient.**
	88.01 88.02 88.03	Tong Guan Tong Shan Tong Tian	Penetrating Gate Passing Mountain Passing Sky	0.3-0.5 cun 0.5-0.8 cun 0.5-1.0 cun	Perpendicular insertion. (Due to cerebral anemia)
	DT04	Wu Ling	5 Mountain Ranges	Micro-puncture	See section on micro-puncture. Then needle 66.03. The blood pressure will be lowered & the vertigo will stop immediately. (Hypotensive)

85

Tung Acupuncture: A Quick Reference Guide

Indications	Point #	Name Pinyin	Name English	Insertion	Comments
Vision blurred	77.18	Shen Guan	Kidney Gate	0.8-2.5 cun	Perpendicular insertion.
	77.28	Guang Ming	Bright Light	0.5-1.0 cun	
	99.07	Er Bei	Ear Back	Micro-puncture	See section on micro-puncture.
	DT04	Wu Ling	5 Mountain Ranges	Micro-puncture	See section on micro-puncture. (Due to hypertension). Then needle Xiasanhuang (77.17, 77.19, 77.21)
Vision debility	66.11	Huo Ju	Fire Chrysanthemum	0.5-0.8 cun	Horizontal insertion. Use on one side only.
	66.12	Huo San	Fire Scatter	0.5-1.0 cun	**Do not use on pregnant patient.**
Vocal cord nodules & polyps	**99.07**	**Er Bei**	**Ear Back**	**Micro-puncture**	**See section on micro-puncture. Do bilaterally. Midway between 99.02 & 99.08. Same as 88.32.**
Vomiting	**44.07**	**Bei Mian**	**Back Face**	**Micro-puncture**	**See section on micro-puncture.**
	1010.07	**Zong Shu**	**Total Pivot**	**0.1-0.2 cun**	**Insert downward. Most effective with Micro-punctureting with extreme caution. Induced by visceral pressures, ICP, food poisoning, meningitis. Only clinically used point.**
	22.14	San Cha San	Three Jam Three	1.0 – 1.5 cun	Towards the palm.
	33.12	Xin Men	Heart Gate	1.0-1.5 cun	**Heart Gate. Always use left arm.** 1.0-1.5 cun insertion next to the bone. CW twist: for intestinal pain, CCW twist: for chest tension.
	77.08	Si Hua Shang	4 Upper Flowers	3.0-3.5 cun	Perpendicular insertion.
	77.09	Si Hua Zhong	4 Middle Flowers	Micro-puncture	See section on micro-puncture.
	77.13	Si Hua Li	4 Inner Flowers	1.5-2.0 cun	Perpendicular insertion.
	1010.19	Shui Tong	Water Through	0.1-0.5 cun	Horizontal insertion. Bilateral.
	1010.20	Shui Jin	Water Gold	0.1-0.5 cun	
	DT03	Chi Shing	Seven Stars	Micro-puncture	See section on micro-puncture.
	DT04	Wu Ling	5 Mountain Ranges	Micro-puncture	See section on micro-puncture.
Water retention	**88.09**	**Tong Shen**	**Passing Kidney**	**0.3-0.5 cun**	**Perpendicular insertion. Excessive water or fat retention.**
Weakness general	**1010.17**	**Qi Kuai**	**Seven Fastness**	**0.5-1.5 cun**	**Perpendicular insertion.**
	1010.01	Zheng Hui	Uprightness Meeting	0.1-0.3 cun	Horizontal insertion. Add 1010.08. Angle and direction of insertion is anterior to posterior insert 60°-90°.
	1010.02	Zhou Yuan	Prefecture Round	0.1-0.3 cun	Horizontal insertion.
	1010.03	Zhou Kun	Prefecture Elder Brother	0.1-0.3 cun	Horizontal insertion.
	1010.04	Zhou Lun	Prefecture Mountain	0.1-0.3 cun	Horizontal insertion.
Whiplash	**44.02**	**Hou Zhui**	**Back Vertibrae**	**0.3-0.5 cun**	**Perpendicular insertion.**
	44.03	**Shou Ying**	**Head Wisdom**	**0.3-0.5 cun**	
Whole body pain	**88.04**	**Jie Mei Yi**	**First Sister**	**1.5-2.0 cun**	**Perpendicular insertion.**
	1010.22	**Bi Yi**	**Nasal Wing**	**0.1-0.2 cun**	**Perpendicular insertion.**
Wound, delayed healing	**44.05**	**Hou Zhi**	**Back Branch**	**0.3-0.7 cun**	**Perpendicular insertion. Add 11.26.**

86

Indications	Point #	Name Pinyin	Name English	Insertion	Comments
Wrist pain	**44.17** **66.16**	**Shui Yu** **Da Zhong**	**Water Cure** **Large Bell**	**0.3-0.5 cun** **1.0-1.5 cun**	**Perpendicular insertion. With cuts, add 11.26 with needle, not micropuncture. (Carple tunnel, arthritis and the like)**
	66.16	**Da Zhong**	**Large Bell**	**1.0-1.5 cun**	**Perpendicular insertion.**
	88.12	**Ming Huang**	**Bright Yellow**	**1.5-2.5 cun**	**Perpendicular insertion. Bilateral.**
	22.08 22.09	Wan shun Yi Wan Shun Er	Wrist Flow One Wrist Flow Two	1.0-1.5 cun 1.0-1.5 cun	Perpendicular insertion.
	77.22	Ce San Li	Lateral 3 Mile	0.5-1.0 cun	Perpendicular insertion. Ipsilateral.
	77.22 77.23	Ce San Li Ce Xia San Li	Lateral 3 Mile Below Lateral 3 Mile	0.5-1.0 cun 0.5-1.0 cun	Perpendicular insertion.
Xerophthalmia	**11.17**	**Mu**	**Wood**	**0.25 cun**	**Shallow insertion, but still touch periosteum. Pinch point before insertion b/c painful.**
Zygomatic pain	22.09	Wan Shun Er	Wrist Flow Two	1.0-1.5 cun	Perpendicular insertion.
	77.07 77.22 77.23	San Zhong Ce San Li Ce Xia San Li	Third Weight Lateral 3 Mile Below Lateral 3 Mile	Micro-puncture 0.5-1.0 cun 0.5-1.0 cun	See section on micro-puncture. Micro-puncture 77.07. Perpendicular insertion 77.22 & 77.23.

Notes:

87

Notes:

Tung Acupuncture

Point Indications
Listed
Numerically

Point	Name Pinyin	English Name	Indications	Insertion
11.01	Da Jian	Big Distance	Coronary artery disease	0.2-0.3 cun
			Inguinal Hernia	
			Knee pain, anterior	
			Opthalmalgia	
			Testitis	
11.02	Xiao Jian	Small Distance	Chronic Bronchitis	0.2-0.3 cun
			Dyspnoea	
			Inguinal Hernia	
			Irritable Heart Syndrome	
			Knee pain, anterior	
			Knee pain	
			Opthalmalgia	
			Palpitations	
			Testitis	
11.03	Fu Jian	Floating Distance	Hernia pain	0.1-0.2 cun
			Inguinal Hernia	
			Stomachache	
			Testitis	
			Toothache	
			Urethritis	
11.04	Wai Jian	External Distance	Hernia pain	0.1-0.2 cun
			Inguinal Hernia	
			Stomachache	
			Toothache	
			Urethritis	
11.05	Zhong Jian	Center Distance	Chest stuffiness	0.2-0.3 cun
			Dizziness	0.2-0.3 cun
			Inguinal Hernia	0.2-0.3 cun
			Knee joint pain	0.2-0.3 cun
			Knee pain, anterior	0.2-0.3 cun
			Palpitations	0.2-0.3 cun
			Testitis	0.2-0.3 cun

Notes:

Point	Name Pinyin	English Name	Indications	Insertion
11.06	Huan Chao	Return Nest	Cervicitis	0.3 cun
			Dysmenorrhea	0.3 cun
			Fallopian tube blockage	0.3 cun
			Frequency miscarriage.	0.3 cun
			Frequent urination	0.3 cun
			Hysteromyoma	0.3 cun
			Infertility	0.3 cun
			Infertilty chronic	0.3 cun
			Inflammation	0.3 cun
			Irregular menstruation	0.3 cun
			Leucorrhea wth reddish discharge	0.3 cun
			Ovarian duct obstruction	0.3 cun
			Polyuria	0.3 cun
			Pudendum swelling	0.3 cun
			Retro version of uterus	0.3 cun
			Uterine myoma	0.3 cun
			Uterine pain	0.3 cun
			Uterine tumor	0.3 cun
			Uteritis	0.3 cun
			Uvulitis	0.3 cun
			Vaginal swelling	0.3 cun
11.07	Zhi Si Ma	Finger 4 Horse	Acne vulgaris	0.1 cun
			Dermatitis, contact	0.1 cun
			Nasal diseases	0.1 cun
			Occipitalgia	0.1 cun
			Pleuritis	0.1 cun
			Rhinitis	0.1 cun
			Rib pain	0.1 cun
			Tinnitus	0.1 cun
11.08	Zhi Wu Jin	Finger 5 Gold	Abdominal pain	0.2-0.3 cun
			Enteritis	0.2-0.3 cun
			Irritable colon	0.2-0.3 cun
11.09	Xin Xi	Heart Knee	Knee pain, anterior	0.1 cun
			Scapulalgia	0.1 cun
			Scapular pain	0.1 cun
11.10	Mu Huo	Wood Fire	Hemiplegia	0.1 cun
11.11	Fei Xin	Lung Heart	Calf muscle pain	0.1 cun
			Lower leg muscle pain	0.1 cun
			Neck pain	0.1 cun
			Spondylaglia	0.1 cun
11.12	Er Jiao Ming	Two Corner Bright	Lower back pain	0.1 cun
			Lumbago	0.1 cun
			Lumbar sprain (Acute)	0.1 cun
			Lumbar sprain (Acute)	Micro-puncture
			Nasal pain	0.1 cun
			Renal pain	0.1 cun
			Sinus pain (At cartilage & bone)	0.1 cun
			Supraorbital pain	0.1 cun

Point	Name Pinyin	English Name	Indications	Insertion
11.13	Dan	Gall Bladder	GB problems	Micro-puncture
			Hysteria	Micro-puncture
			Knee joint pain	Micro-puncture
			Nocturnal crying (child)	Micro-puncture
			Palpitations	Micro-puncture
11.14	Zhi San Zhong	Finger 3 Layer	Augment breast size	0.1 cun
			Bells palsy	0.1 cun
			Breast augmentation	0.1 cun
			Muscular atrophy Muscular dystrophy	0.1 cun
			Periductal mastitis	0.1 cun
11.15	Zhi Shen	Finger Kidney	Back pain	0.1 cun
			Dry mouth	0.1 cun
			Enragement, Sudden then faint	0.1 cun
			Heart failure	0.1 cun
			Kidney symptoms	0.1 cun
			Low back pain	0.1 cun
			Premature ejaculation	0.1 cun
			Sexual neurosis	0.1 cun
			Thirst	0.1 cun
11.16	Huo Xi	Fire Knee	Arthritis (RA, OA)	0.1 cun
			Knee pain	0.1 cun
			Knee pain, anterior	0.1 cun
			Mitral valve disease	0.1 cun
			Rheumatic heart disease	0.1 cun
11.17	Mu	Wood	Allergy, nasal	0.25 cun
			Bad temper	0.25 cun
			Common cold	0.25 cun
			Contact dermatitis of hands	0.25 cun
			Dry eyes	0.25 cun
			Dryness of the nose	0.25 cun
			Eczema, acute	0.25 cun
			Eye dryness	0.25 cun
			Hernia of the large intestine	0.25 cun
			Hyperactivity of liver-fire and irritability	0.25 cun
			Hyperhydrosis	0.25 cun
			Itching skin	0.25 cun
			Lacrimation due to wind exposure	0.25 cun
			Nasal allergy	0.25 cun
			Nose, running	0.25 cun
			Pruritis	0.25 cun
			Rhinitis, acute	0.25 cun
			Sweating excessive	0.25 cun
			Tinea	0.25 cun
			Xerophthalmia	0.25 cun
11.18	Pi Zhong	Spleen Edema	Myoplastic anemia	0.1 cun
			Splenitis	0.1 cun
			Splenomegaly	0.1 cun
			Splenopathy	0.1 cun

93

Point	Name Pinyin	English Name	Indications	Insertion
11.19	Xin Chang	Heart Normal	Ankle pain	0.1-0.2 cun
			Bradicardia	0.1-0.2 cun
			Cardiac arrhythmias	0.1-0.2 cun
			Heart beat (Abnormal)	0.1-0.2 cun
			Palpitations	0.1-0.2 cun
			Rheumatic heart disease	0.1-0.2 cun
			Tachycardia	0.1-0.2 cun
11.20	Mu Yan	Wood Inflammation	Hepatitis A	0.2 cun
			Hepatomegaly	0.2 cun
			Liver cirrhosis	0.2 cun
11.21	San Yan	Three Eyes	Fatigue	0.2 cun
			Lack of energy	0.2 cun
11.22	Fu Yuan	Recover	Rheumatoid arthritis	0.1 cun
11.23	Yan Huang	Eye Yellow	Eye jaundice	0.2 cun
			Hepatitis	0.2 cun
11.24	Fu Ke	Lady Class	Abdominal distension (Cyst indigestion)	0.2 cun
			Distension of the lower abdomen	0.2 cun
			Dysmenorrhea	0.2 cun
			Female sterility	0.2 cun
			Gynecological, problems	0.2 cun
			Hysteroma	0.2 cun
			Hysteromyoma	0.2 cun
			Infertilty chronic	0.2 cun
			Infertility	0.2 cun
			Irregular menstruation	0.2 cun
			Leucorrhea with red & white discharge	0.2 cun
			Menorrhagia	0.2 cun
			Oligo menorrhea	0.2 cun
			Ovarian duct obstruction	0.2 cun
			Pain of uterus (Acute or chronic)	0.2 cun
			Premenstrual tension syndrome	0.2 cun
			Pudendum swelling	0.2 cun
			Scanty menstruation	0.2 cun
			Uterine tumor	0.2 cun
			Uterismus (Uterus pain)	0.2 cun
			Uteritis	0.2 cun
			Vaginitis	0.2 cun
11.25	Zhi Xian	Stop Saliva	Ptyalism	0.2 cun
11.26	Zhi Wu	Control Dirt	Abscess	Micro-puncture
			Bed sore	Micro-puncture
			Blood oozing from the wound after a surgery	Micro-puncture
			Delayed bone healing	Micro-puncture
			Delayed wound healing	Micro-puncture
			Herpes zoster	Micro-puncture
			Otitis media	Micro-puncture
			Persisted carbuncles	Micro-puncture
			Poor wound healing	Micro-puncture

Point	Name Pinyin	English Name	Indications	Insertion
11.27	Wu Hu	Five Tigers	Ankle pain	0.2 cun
			Ankle sprain	0.2 cun
			Bone swelling of all body	0.2 cun
			Finger joint pain	0.2 cun
			Finger numbness	0.2 cun
			Finger pain index finger	0.2 cun
			Foot pain	0.2 cun
			Foot pain (Dorsal)	0.2 cun
			Gout	0.2 cun
			Headache: Frontal	0.2 cun
			Heel pain	0.2 cun
			Heel pain	0.2 cun
			Joint pain all	0.2 cun
			Joint swelling	0.2 cun
			Osteoarthritis	0.2 cun
			Pain in the heel	0.2 cun
			Pain of the finger joints	0.2 cun
			Rheumatoid arthritis	0.2 cun
			Shoulder-arm pain	0.2 cun
			Sports injury	0.2 cun
			Tenosynovitis	0.2 cun
			Toe numbness	0.2 cun
			Toe pain	0.2 cun
			Toe pain due to gout	0.2 cun
11.28	Bei Tong	Back Pain	Scapular pain	0.1 cun
			Scapular pain	0.1 cun
11.29	Lao Hu	A Tiger	Ankle pain	0.1 cun

Notes:

95

Tung Acupuncture: A Quick Reference Guide

Point	Name Pinyin	English Name	Indications	Insertion
22.01	Zhong Zi	Double Son	Acromion pain	1.0-1.5 cun
			Asthmatic breathing	1.0-1.5 cun
			Back ache (Bilateral)	1.0-1.5 cun
			Back ache (Unilateral)	1.0-1.5 cun
			Back ache to shoulder	1.0-1.5 cun
			Back pain	1.0-1.5 cun
			Backache along UB meridian	1.0-1.5 cun
			Bronchial asthma (Esp. for children)	1.0-1.5cun
			Chest & back pain	1.0-1.5 cun
			Common cold	1.0-1.5 cun
			COPD Atelectasis.	1.0-1.5 cun
			Coughing and asthma (Most effective with children)	1.0-1.5 cun
			Hand pain difficulty holding object	1.0-1.5 cun
			Hand spasm Tendon issue	1.0-1.5 cun
			Hemiplegia	1.0-1.5 cun
			Hysteromyoma	1.0-1.5 cun
			Influenza	1.0-1.5cun
			Knee joint pain	1.0-1.5 cun
			Neck sprain	1.0-1.5 cun
			Pain of the acromion	1.0-1.5 cun
			Pneumonia	1.0-1.5 cun
			Scapular muscle pain	1.0-1.5cun
			Scapular pain	1.0-1.5 cun
			Shoulder & back pain	1.0-1.5 cun
			Spasm of the hand tendon issue	1.0-1.5 cun
			Sprain neck	1.0-1.5 cun
			Stroke with hand convulsions	1.0-1.5 cun
22.02	Zhong Xian	Double Saint	Acromion pain	1.0-1.5 cun
			Asthmatic breathing	1.0-1.5 cun
			Back ache (Bilateral)	1.0-1.5 cun
			Back ache (Unilateral)	1.0-1.5 cun
			Back ache to neck	1.0-1.5 cun
			Back pain	1.0-1.5 cun
			Backache along UB meridian	1.0-1.5 cun
			Chest & back pain	1.0-1.5 cun
			Fever, high	1.0-1.5cun
			Hand pain difficulty holding object	1.0-1.5 cun
			Hand spasm Tendon issue	1.0-1.5 cun
			Hemiplegia	1.0-1.5 cun
			High fever	1.0-1.5 cun
			Hysteromyoma	1.0-1.5 cun
			Knee joint pain	1.0-1.5 cun
			Knee pain	1.0-1.5 cun
			Knee pain, anterior	1.0-1.5cun
			Pain of the acromion	1.0-1.5 cun
			Pneumonia	1.0-1.5 cun
			Spasm of the hand tendon issue	1.0-1.5 cun
			Stroke with hand convulsions	1.0-1.5 cun

Tung Acupuncture: A Quick Reference Guide

Point	Name Pinyin	English Name	Indications	Insertion
22.03	Shang Bai	Upper White	Angina pectoris	0.3-0.5 cun
			Chest & back pain	0.3-0.5 cun
			Chest pain	0.3-0.5 cun
			Conjunctivitis	0.3-0.5 cun
			Eye, red	0.3-0.5 cun
			Impact injury	0.3-0.5 cun
			Neck sprain	0.3-0.5 cun
			Sciatica	0.3-0.5 cun
22.04	Da Bai	Big White	Asthma (In children)	Deep insert to 2.01
			Asthmatic breathing	Micro-puncture
			Back pain	Deep insert to 2.01
			Fever, High	Micro-puncture
			Headache	Deep insert to 2.01
			Headache Due to common cold	Deep insert to 2.01
			Hemiplegia	Deep insert to 2.01
			High Fever (Most effective)	Micro-puncture
			Insomnia	Deep insert to 2.01
			Low back pain	Deep insert to 2.01
			Pneumonia	Micro-puncture
			Sciatica	Deep insert to 2.01
			Sciatica Due to lung deficiency	Deep insert to 2.01

Notes:

Point	Name Pinyin	English Name	Indications	Insertion
22.05	Ling Gu	Androit Bone	Abdominal distension Lower	Deep insert to 2.02
			Abdominal pain	Deep insert to 2.02
			Abdominal pain & distension (Lower)	Deep insert to 2.02
			Amenorrhea	Deep insert to 2.02
			Back pain	Deep insert to 2.02
			Bells palsy (Facial nerve palsy)	Deep insert to 2.02
			Bone diseases	Deep insert to 2.02
			Coma	Deep insert to 2.02
			Difficult delivery	Deep insert to 2.02
			Elbow joint pain	Deep insert to 2.02
			Headache	Deep insert to 2.02
			Hearing impairment	Deep insert to 2.02
			Heel pain	Deep insert to 2.02
			Hemiplegia	Deep insert to 2.02
			Joint pain	Deep insert to 2.02
			Leg pain	Deep insert to 2.02
			Low back pain	Deep insert to 2.02
			Low back pain (Acute sprain)	Deep insert to 2.02
			Lumbago	Deep insert to 2.02
			Meniere's Syndrome	Deep insert to 2.02
			Menorrhea	Deep insert to 2.02
			Migraine	Deep insert to 2.02
			Pain in the heel	Deep insert to 2.02
			Polyuria	Deep insert to 2.02
			Poor appetite	Deep insert to 2.02
			Qi deficiency	Deep insert to 2.02
			Sciatica	Deep insert to 2.02
			Sciatica Due to lung deficiency	Deep insert to 2.02
			Spinal pain	Deep insert to 2.02
			Stye	Deep insert to 2.02
			Tendon diseases	Deep insert to 2.02
			Tinnitus	Deep insert to 2.02
			Toothache	Deep insert to 2.02
			Vertigo	Deep insert to 2.02

Notes:

Point	Name Pinyin	English Name	Indications	Insertion
22.06	Zhong Bai	Center White	Ankle injury (External ligament)	0.3-0.5 cun
			Ankle pain	0.3-0.5 cun
			Astigmatism	0.3-0.5 cun
			Back pain	0.3-0.5 cun
			Back pain (Bilateral)	0.3-0.5 cun
			Biliary ascariasis	0.3-0.5 cun
			Biliary colic	0.3-0.5 cun
			Bone swelling	0.3-0.5 cun
			Dizziness	0.3-0.5 cun
			Ear distension	0.3-0.5 cun
			Edema	0.3-0.5 cun
			Fatigue	0.3-0.5 cun
			Hypertension	Micro-puncture
			Low back pain	0.3-0.5 cun
			Lower back pain due to Kidney deficiency	0.3-0.5 cun
			Lumbago	0.3-0.5 cun
			Neck sprain	0.3-0.5 cun
			Nephritis	0.3-0.5 cun
			Nephrosis	0.3-0.5 cun
			Osteoarthritis	0.3-0.5 cun
			Sciatica	0.3-0.5 cun
			Umbilical pain	0.3-0.5 cun
22.07	Xia Bai	Lower White	Ankle injury (External ligament)	0.3-0.5 cun
			Astigmatism	0.3-0.5 cun
			Back pain	0.3-0.5 cun
			Back pain (Bilateral)	0.3-0.5 cun
			Biliary ascariasis	0.3-0.5 cun
			Biliary colic	0.3-0.5 cun
			Bone swelling	0.3-0.5 cun
			Cholecystitis	0.3-0.5 cun
			Cholic pain due to renal stones	0.3-0.5 cun
			Dizziness	0.3-0.5 cun
			Edema	0.3-0.5 cun
			Fainting during acupuncture	0.3-0.5 cun
			Fatigue	0.3-0.5 cun
			Hypertension	0.3-0.5 cun
			Kidney diseases	0.3-0.5 cun
			Low back pain	0.3-0.5 cun
			Lumbago	0.3-0.5 cun
			Myopia	0.3-0.5 cun
			Nephritis	0.3-0.5 cun
			Nephrosis	0.3-0.5 cun
			Osteoarthritis	0.3-0.5 cun
			Pain in the heel	0.3-0.5 cun
			Renal calculus with renal colic pain	0.3-0.5 cun
			Renal colic	0.3-0.5 cun
			Renal stones cholic pain	0.3-0.5 cun
			Sciatica	0.3-0.5 cun
			Umbilical pain	0.3-0.5 cun

Tung Acupuncture: A Quick Reference Guide

Point	Name Pinyin	English Name	Indications	Insertion
22.08	Wan Shun Yi	Wrist Flow One	Abdominal distension Lower	1.0-1.5 cun
			Back pain	1.0-1.5 cun
			Back pain (Bilateral)	1.0-1.5 cun
			Blurred vision	1.0-1.5 cun
			Bone swelling in all extremities	1.0-1.5 cun
			Cervical bone spurs with hand numbness	1.0-1.5 cun
			Epilepsy	1.0-1.5 cun
			Eye problems	1.0-1.5 cun
			Eye twitching	1.0-1.5 cun
			Facial spasm	1.0-1.5 cun
			Fatigue	1.0-1.5 cun
			Golfers elbow	1.0-1.5 cun
			Headache	1.0-1.5 cun
			Heavy para-spinal pain (low back)	1.0-1.5 cun
			Kidney Deficiency Syndrome	1.0-1.5 cun
			Lower back pain due to Kidney deficiency	1.0-1.5 cun
			Myopia	1.0-1.5 cun
			Nephritis (Acute or chronic)	1.0-1.5 cun
			Pain of the wrist joint	1.0-1.5 cun
			Sciatica	1.0-1.5 cun
			Spinal sprain acute	1.0-1.5 cun
			Spinal vertebrae spur	1.0-1.5 cun
			Tinnitus	1.0-1.5 cun
			Tiredness	1.0-1.5 cun
			Twitching of the eye	1.0-1.5 cun
			Umbilical pain	1.0-1.5 cun
			Wrist joint pain	1.0-1.5 cun
22.09	Wan Shun Er	Wrist Flow Two	Abdominal distension Lower	1.0-1.5 cun
			Back pain	1.0-1.5 cun
			Low back pain	1.0-1.5 cun
			Blurred vision	1.0-1.5 cun
			Bone swelling in all extremities	1.0-1.5 cun
			Epilepsy	1.0-1.5 cun
			Eye twitching	1.0-1.5 cun
			Facial spasm	1.0-1.5 cun
			Fatigue	1.0-1.5 cun
			Headache	1.0-1.5 cun
			Heavy para-spinal pain (low back and back)	1.0-1.5 cun
			Kidney Deficiency Syndrome	1.0-1.5 cun
			Nephritis (Acute or chronic)	1.0-1.5 cun
			Pain of the wrist joint	1.0-1.5 cun
			Sciatica	1.0-1.5 cun
			Tinnitus	1.0-1.5 cun
			Tiredness	1.0-1.5 cun
			Twitching of the eye	1.0-1.5 cun
			Umbilical pain	1.0-1.5 cun
			Wrist joint pain	1.0-1.5 cun
			Epistaxis	1.0-1.5 cun
			Hip pain	1.0-1.5 cun
			Zygomatic pain	1.0-1.5 cun

100

© Theodore L. Zombolas PhD (AM), LAc, Dipl.Ac. (NCCAOM). ©

Point	Name Pinyin	English Name	Indications	Insertion
22.10	Shou Jie	Hand Release	Fainting during acupuncture	0.5 cun
			Syncope, iatrogenic	0.5 cun
22.11	Tu Shui	Earth Water	Asthmatic breathing	0.2-0.3 cun
			Duodenal ulcer	0.2-0.3 cun
			Gastric ulcer	0.2-0.3 cun
			Phalangitis	0.2-0.3 cun
			Pneumonia	0.2-0.3 cun
			Stomach ache (Acute)	0.2-0.3 cun
			Throat Sore	0.2-0.3 cun
22.12	San Cha Yi	Three Jam One	Lung diseases	1.0 – 1.5 cun
22.13	San Cha Er	Three Jam Two	Leg pain (Anterior Tibia, shin plints, compartment syndrome)	1.0–1.5 cun
22.14	San Cha San	Three Jam Three	Allergic rhinitis	1.0 – 1.5 cun
			Allergies: Itching of skin due to allergies	1.0 – 1.5 cun
			Back pain low	1.0 – 1.5 cun
			Bone Swelling	1.0 – 1.5 cun
			Common cold	1.0 – 1.5 cun
			Earache	1.0 – 1.5 cun
			Eyes, difficulty opening	1.0 – 1.5 cun
			Fatigue	1.0 – 1.5 cun
			Headache	1.0 – 1.5 cun
			Hypochondriac pain	1.0 – 1.5 cun
			Itching of skin due to allergies	1.0 – 1.5 cun
			Low back pain	1.0 – 1.5 cun
			Mypoia	1.0 – 1.5 cun
			Nausea	1.0 – 1.5 cun
			Neck sprain	1.0 – 1.5 cun
			Pain of the thigh	1.0 – 1.5 cun
			Palpitations	1.0 – 1.5 cun
			Shoulder pain	1.0 – 1.5 cun
			Sprain neck	1.0 – 1.5 cun
			Tachycardia	1.0 – 1.5 cun
			Thigh pain	1.0 – 1.5 cun
			Thigh pain and soreness	1.0 – 1.5 cun
			Throat Sore	1.0 – 1.5 cun
			Tinnitus	1.0 – 1.5 cun
			Toothache	1.0 – 1.5 cun
			Vomiting	1.0 – 1.5 cun
22.15	Xi Gai	Knee	Knee pain	0.5-1.0 cun
22.16	Wan Bing	10,000 Maladies	Panacea for diseases	0.5 cun
33.01	Qi Men	This Door	Anal prolapse	0.2-0.5 cun
			Hemorrhoid pain (Internal external)	0.2-0.5 cun
			Leucorrhea	0.2-0.5 cun
33.02	Qi Jiao	This Corner	Hemorrhoid pain (Internal external)	0.2-0.5 cun
			Leucorrhea	0.2-0.5 cun
			Menorrhea hyper-Oligo	0.2-0.5 cun
33.03	Qi Zheng	This Uprightness	Anal prolapse	0.2-0.5 cun
			Hemorrhoid pain (Internal external)	0.2-0.5 cun
			Leucorrhea	0.2-0.5 cun

Point	Name Pinyin	English Name	Indications	Insertion
33.04	Hou Chuan	Fire Threaded	Arm pain (Forearm)	0.3-0.5 cun
			Constipation	0.3-0.5 cun
			Forearm pain/cramp	0.3-0.5 cun
			Palpitations	0.3-0.5 cun
			Sciatica	0.3-0.5 cun
33.05	Huo Ling	Fire Mound	Sciatica	0.5-1.0 cun
			Arm cramp	0.5-1.0 cun
			Chest pain	0.5-1.0 cun
			Chest pain (Heart problem)	0.5-1.0 cun
			Chest stuffiness	0.5-1.0 cun
			Forearm pain/cramp	0.5-1.0 cun
			Sciatica	0.5-1.0 cun
33.06	Huo Shan	Fire Mountain	Chest pain (Heart problem)	1.0-1.5 cun
			Chest stuffiness	1.0-1.5 cun
			Cramping o the hand and arm	1.0-1.5 cun
			Forearm pain/cramp	1.0-1.5 cun
			Sciatica	1.0-1.5 cun
33.07	Huo Fu Hai	Fire Bowels	Anemia	0.5-1.0 cun
			Asthma	0.5-1.0 cun
			Chronic Fatigue	0.5-1.0 cun.
			Common cold	0.5-1.0 cun
			Cough	0.5-1.0 cun
			Dyspnoea	0.5-1.0 cun
			Elbow joint pain	0.5-1.0 cun
			Nasal obstruction	0.5-1.0 cun
			Rhinitis	0.5-1.0 cun
			Sciatica	0.5-1.0 cun
33.08	Shou Wu Jin	Hand Five Gold	Abdominal pain	0.3-0.5 cun
			Calf pain	0.3-0.5 cun
			Foot pain (Dorsal)	0.3-0.5 cun
			Leg pain	0.3-0.5 cun
			Nerve impingement	0.3-0.5 cun
			Neuralgia	0.3-0.5 cun
			Sciatica	0.3-0.5 cun
			Tarsal tunnel	0.3-0.5 cun
33.09	Shou Qian Jin	Hand 1000 Gold	Abdominal pain	0.3-0.5 cun
			Calf pain	0.3-0.5 cun
			Leg pain	0.3-0.5 cun
			Nerve impingement	0.3-0.5 cun
			Neuralgia	0.3-0.5 cun
			Sciatica	0.3-0.5 cun
			Tarsal tunnel	0.3-0.5 cun

Notes:

Point	Name Pinyin	English Name	Indications	Insertion
33.10	Chang Men	Intestine Gate	Blurred vision	1.0-1.5 cun
			Colitis (LI)	1.0-1.5 cun
			Diarrhea acute	1.0-1.5 cun
			Dizziness	1.0-1.5 cun
			Enteritis (SI)	1.0-1.5 cun
			Enteritis acute	1.0-1.5 cun
			Enteritis caused by hepatitis	1.0-1.5 cun
			Enteritis chronic	1.0-1.5 cun
			Giddiness (Metabolic impairment)	1.0-1.5 cun
			Hepatitis acute	1.0-1.5 cun
			Large intestine distending pain	1.0-1.5 cun
			Proctitis (Rectum)	1.0-1.5 cun
33.11	Gan Men	Liver Gate	Aplastic anemia	1.0-1.5 cun
			Chest tension	1.0-1.5 cun
			Cramp of the foot	1.0-1.5 cun
			Erythropenia	1.0-1.5 cun
			Foot cramp	1.0-1.5 cun
			Hepatitis	1.0-1.5 cun
			Hepatitis acute	1.0-1.5 cun
			Intestine Pain.	1.0-1.5 cun
			Jaundice	1.0-1.5 cun
			Jaundice due to acute Hepatitis	1.0-1.5 cun
			Leucopenia	1.0-1.5 cun
			Liver GB diseases	1.0-1.5 cun
33.12	Xin Men	Heart Gate	Bradicardia	1.0-1.5 cun
			Cardiac arrhythmias	1.0-1.5 cun
			Carditis	1.0-1.5 cun
			Chest oppression	1.0-1.5 cun
			Coccyx pain	1.0-1.5 cun
			Golfers elbow	1.0-1.5 cun
			Groin pain region	1.0-1.5 cun
			Hip pain	1.0-1.5 cun
			Inguinal pain (Due to ishemia)	1.0-1.5 cun
			Knee joint pain	1.0-1.5 cun
			Myocarditis	1.0-1.5 cun
			Palpitations	1.0-1.5 cun
			Stomach distension	1.0-1.5 cun
			Tachycardia	1.0-1.5 cun
			Vomiting	1.0-1.5 cun
33.13	Ren Shi	Human Scholar	Asthma (Adult) Acute or chronic	0.5-1.0 cun
			Back pain	0.5-1.0 cun
			Finger joint pain	0.5-1.0 cun
			Finger pain	0.5-1.0 cun
			Hand pain (Flexor tendonitis, palm side)	0.5-1.0 cun
			Pain of the finger joints	0.5-1.0 cun
			Palm pain	0.5-1.0 cun
			Shoulder frozen	0.5-1.0 cun
			Shoulder pain syndrome (Any pain from shoulder to wrist & scapula)	0.5-1.0 cun

103

Point	Name Pinyin	English Name	Indications	Insertion
33.14	Di Shi	Earth Scholar	Angina pectoris	1.0-1.5 cun
			Asthma (Adult) Acute or chronic	1.0-1.5 cun
			Chest pain	1.0-1.5 cun
			Common cold	1.0-1.5 cun.
			Headache	1.0-1.5 cun
			Neurosis	1.0-1.5 cun
33.15	Tian Shi	Heaven Scholar	Arm pain	1.0-1.5 cun
			Arm pain (Upper)	1.0-1.5 cun
			Asthma (Adult) Acute or chronic	1.0-1.5 cun
			Common cold	1.0-1.5 cun
			Dyspnoea	1.0-1.5 cun
			Rhinitis	1.0-1.5 cun
33.16	Qu Ling	Curved Mound	Abdominal pain lower	Micro-puncture
			Arthritis (Esp. elbow)	0.3-0.5 cun
			Asthma	0.3-0.5 cun
			Asthmatic breathing	Micro-puncture
			Cardiac arrest	Micro-puncture
			Ear distension	0.3-0.5 cun
			Frozen shoulder	0.3-0.5 cun
			Gastro-enteritis	Micro-puncture
			Hand spasm tendon issue	0.3-0.5 cun
			Heart palpitations	Micro-puncture
			Muscle spasm	0.3-0.5 cun
			Palpitations	Micro-puncture
			Pneumonia	Micro-puncture
			Shoulder difficlty lifting	0.3-0.5 cun
			Spasm of the hand tendon issue	0.3-0.5 cun
			Stroke with hand convulsions	Micro-puncture
			Tinnitus	0.3-0.5 cun
44.01	Fen Jin	Dividing Gold	Common cold	0.5-1.0 cun
			Rhinitis	0.5-1.0 cun
44.02	Hou Zhui	Back Vertibrae	Cervical spine issues	0.3-0.5 cun
			Disc prolapse	0.3-0.5 cun
			Hypertension	0.3-0.5 cun
			Lumbago	0.3-0.5 cun
			Nephritis (HTN)	0.3-0.5 cun
			Spinal pain	0.3-0.5 cun
			Whiplash	0.3-0.5 cun
44.03	Shou Ying	Head Wisdom	Disc prolapse	0.3-0.5 cun
			Hypertension	0.3-0.5 cun
			Lumbago	0.3-0.5 cun
			Nephritis (HTN)	0.3-0.5 cun
			Slipped disc	0.3-0.5 cun
			Spinal pain	0.3-0.5 cun
			Whiplash	0.3-0.5 cun

Notes:

Point	Name Pinyin	English Name	Indications	Insertion
44.04	Fu Ding	Wealth Summit	Arteriosclerosis	0.5 cun
			Cholesterol	0.5 cun
			Dizziness	0.5 cun
			Facial paralysis	0.5 cun
			Fatigue	0.3 cun
			Headache	0.5 cun
			Hypertension	0.5 cun
			Neck pain	0.5 cun
44.05	Hou Zhi	Back Branch	Arteriosclerosis	0.3-0.7 cun
			Cholesterol	0.3-0.7 cun
			Delayed wound healing	0.3-0.7 cun
			Dizziness	0.3-0.7 cun
			Facial paralysis	0.3-0.7 cun
			Headache	0.3-0.7 cun
			Hypertension	0.3-0.7 cun
			Neck pain	0.3-0.7 cun
			Skin diseases (All major)	0.3-0.7 cun
			Wound, delayed healing	0.3-0.7 cun
44.06	Jian Zhong	Shoulder Center	Arteriosclerosis	1.0-1.5 cun
			Dysuria	1.0-1.5 cun
			Epistaxis	1.0-1.5 cun
			Frozen shoulder	1.0-1.5 cun
			Hemiplegia	1.0-1.5 cun
			Knee joint pain	1.0-1.5 cun
			Knee pain	1.0-1.5 cun
			Knee pain cold	1.0-1.5 cun
			Leg numbness	1.0-1.5 cun
			Leg pain cold	1.0-1.5 cun
			Leg weakness	1.0-1.5 cun
			Nasal bleeding	1.0-1.5 cun
			Nasal obstruction with common cold	1.0-1.5 cun
			Poliomyelitis (Infantile paralysis)	0.5-1.0 cun
			Shoulder joint sprain	1.0-1.5 cun
			Shoulder pain	1.0-1.5 cun
			Shoulder problems	1.0-1.5 cun
			Shoulder-hand pain	1.0-1.5 cun
			Skin disorder (Esp. neck skin)	1.0-1.5 cun
			Thigh pain and soreness	1.0-1.5 cun
			Tongue rigidity (Aphasia due to apoplexy)	1.0-1.5 cun
			Urticaria on upper part of the body	1.0-1.5 cun
44.07	Bei Mian	Back Face	Abdominal distension	0.3-0.5 cun
			Enteritis, Acute and chronic	Micro-puncture
			Food poisoning acute	0.3-0.5 cun
			Hoarseness	0.3-0.5 cun
			Laryngitis	0.3-0.5 cun
			Leg muscle pain	Micro-puncture
			Thigh pain and soreness	Micro-puncture
			Tiredness	Micro-puncture
			Vomiting	Micro-puncture

Point	Name Pinyin	English Name	Indications	Insertion
44.08	Ren Zong	Man Ancestor	Arm pain	Micro-puncture
			Asthma	0.5 cun
			Cardiac diseases	0.8 cun
			Common cold	0.5 cun
			Foot pain	1.2 cun
			Jaundice	1.2 cun
			Peripheral edema (K failure)	0.8 cun
			Spleen enlargement	1.2 cun
			Splenomegaly	1.2 cun
44.09	Di Zong	Earth Ancestor	Angina pectoris	1.0-2.0 cun
			Arteriosclerosis	1.0-2.0 cun
			Cardiac arrest	1.0-2.0 cun
			Coronary artery disease	1.0-2.0 cun
			Shock (most important point)	1.0-2.0 cun
44.10	Tian Zong	Heaven Ancestor	Angina pectoris	1.0-1.5 cun
			Body odor	1.0-1.5 cun
			Bromhidrosis	1.0-1.5 cun
			Cardiac diseases	1.0-1.5 cun
			Diabetes mellitus	1.0-1.5 cun
			Groin pain	1.0-1.5 cun
			Leg pain	1.0-1.5 cun
			Leucorrhea	1.0-1.5 cun
			Poliomyelitis (Muscle atrophy)	1.0-1.5 cun
			Vaginitis (Tenderness & pruritis)	1.0-1.5 cun
44.11	Yun Bai	Cloud White	Dysuria	0.3-0.5 cun
			Knee joint pain	0.3-0.5 cun
			Leucorrhea	0.3-0.5 cun
			Poliomyelitis (Muscle atrophy)	0.3-0.5 cun
			Vaginitis	0.3-0.5 cun
44.12	Li Bai	Plum White	Armpit odor	0.5 cun
			Bromhidrosis	0.5 cun
			Feet pain	0.5 cun
			Knee pain	0.5 cun
			Leg pain	0.5 cun
			Poliomyelitis (Lower extremities muscle wasting)	0.5 cun
44.13	Zhi Tong	Branch Through	Arteriosclerosis	1.0 cun
			Back pain low	1.0 cun
			Dizziness	1.0 cun
			Fatigue	1.0 cun
			Hypertension	1.0 cun
			Low back pain	1.0 cun
44.14	Luo Tong	Drop Through	Arteriosclerosis	0.6-1.0 cun
			Back pain low	0.6-1.0 cun
			Dizziness	0.6-1.0 cun
			Fatigue	0.6-1.0 cun
			Hypertension	0.6-1.0 cun

Tung Acupuncture: A Quick Reference Guide

Point	Name Pinyin	English Name	Indications	Insertion
44.15	Xia Qu	Lower Curve	Dysuria	0.6-1.0 cun
			Hemiplegia	0.6-1.0 cun
			Hypertension	0.6-1.0 cun
			Poliomyelitis	0.6-1.0 cun
			Sciatica	0.6-1.0 cun
			Sulaxation of joint (Due to falls and accident)	0.6-1.0 cun
44.16	Shang Qu	Upper Curve	Arm pain	0.6-1.5 cun
			Cirrhosis	Micro-puncture
			Hypertension	0.6-1.5 cun
			Knee pain	0.6-1.5 cun
			Leg pain	0.6-1.5 cun
			Liver GB diseases	Micro-puncture
			Poliomyelitis	0.6-1.5 cun
			Sciatica	0.6-1.5 cun
44.17	Shui Yu	Water Cure	Arm pain	Micro-puncture
			Knee joint pain	0.3-0.5 cun
			Leg muscle pain	0.3-0.5 cun
			Lumbago	0.3-0.5 cun
			Nephritis (Protein urea)	Micro-puncture
			Protein urea	Micro-puncture
			Renal stone	Micro-puncture
			Wrist pain (Carple tunnel, arthritis and the like)	0.3-0.5 cun
55.01	Huo Bao	Fire Bag	Alcohol intoxication	0.3-0.5 cun
			Angina pectoris	0.3-0.5 cun
			Cardiac arrest	Micro-puncture
			Labor difficulty	0.3-0.5 cun
			Placenta retention	0.3-0.5 cun
55.02	Hua Gu Yi	Flower Bone 1	Blepharitis (Eyelid inflammation)	0.5-1.0 cun
			Conjunctivitis	0.5-1.0 cun
			Deafness	0.5-1.0 cun
			Headache (Mainly frontal)	0.5-1.0 cun
			Loss of hearing	0.5-1.0 cun
			Nasal pain	0.5-1.0 cun
			Ophthalmia	0.5-1.0 cun
			Photophobia	0.5-1.0 cun
			Tinnitus	0.5-1.0 cun
			Toothache (Upper & lower)	0.5-1.0 cun
			Trachoma (Eye infection)	0.5-1.0 cun
55.03	Hua Gu Er	Flower Bone 2	Arm pain (Forearm)	0.5-1.0cun
			Finger weakness (Tremor type weakness, gripping power)	0.5-1.0 cun
			Frozen shoulder	0.5-1.0 cun
			Shoulder difficlty lifting	0.5-1.0 cun
55.04	Hua Gu San	Flower Bone 3	Back pain	0.8 cun
			Sciatica	0.8 cun
			Spinal pain	0.8 cun

107

Point	Name Pinyin	English Name	Indications	Insertion
55.05	Hua Gu Si	Flower Bone 4	Abdominal pain	0.5-1.0 cun
			Haemorrhageic disorders	0.5-1.0 cun
			Purpuras	0.5-1.0 cun
			Sciatica	0.5-1.0 cun
			Spinal pain	0.5-1.0 cun
			Stomach ache	0.5-1.0 cun
			Thrombocytopenia	0.5-1.0 cun
55.06	Shang Liu	Upper Tumor	Cranial nerve Neuralgia	0.3-0.5 cun
			Cranial tumors All types	0.3-0.5 cun
			Epilepsy	0.3-0.5 cun
			Headache	0.3-0.5 cun
			Hydrocephalus	0.3-0.5 cun
			Intentional tremor	0.3-0.5 cun
			Migraine	0.3-0.5 cun
			Palsy	0.3-0.5 cun
			Trigeminal neuralgia	0.3-0.5 cun
66.01	Hai Bao	Seal	Coccyx pain	0.1-0.3 cun
			Conjunctivitis	0.1-0.3 cun
			Frequent urination	0.1-0.3 cun
			Hernia pain	0.1-0.3 cun
			Index finger pain	0.1-0.3 cun
			Inguinal hernia	0.1-0.3 cun
			Myopia	0.1-0.3 cun
			Thumb pain (De Quervain's Tendonitis)	0.1-0.3 cun
			Vaginitis	0.1-0.3 cun
66.02	Mu Fu	Wood Wife	Amenorrhea	0.2-0.4 cun
			Dysmenorrhea	0.2-0.4 cun
			Frequent urination	0.2-0.4 cun
			Infertility	0.2-0.4 cun
			Leucorrhea with red & white discharge	0.2-0.4 cun
			Metritis (Uterine inflammation)	0.2-0.4 cun
			Sterility (Partial obstruction of Fallopian tubes) (Decreased sperm motility)	0.2-0.4 cun
			Uterine inflammation	0.2-0.4 cun

Notes:

Point	Name Pinyin	English Name	Indications	Insertion
66.03	Huo Ying	Fire Hardness	Angina pectoris	0.3-0.5 cun
			Bone swelling	0.3-0.5 cun
			Cardiac arrest	0.3-0.5 cun
			Cardiac diseases	0.3-0.5 cun
			Coma	0.3-0.5 cun
			Dizziness	0.3-0.5 cun
			Dysuria	0.3-0.5 cun
			Giddiness	0.3-0.5 cun
			Glaucoma	0.3-0.5 cun
			Heart paralysis (For resuscitation)	0.3-0.5 cun
			Hypertension	0.3-0.5 cun
			Mandible pain (Difficulty opening mouth)	0.3-0.5 cun
			Metritis (Uterine inflammation)	0.3-0.5 cun
			Mouth (Difficulty opening) mandible pain	0.3-0.5 cun
			Palpitations	0.3-0.5 cun
			Placenta accreta (retention)	0.3-0.5 cun
			Placental dystocia	0.3-0.5 cun
			Pudendum swelling	0.3-0.5 cun
			TMJ pain	0.3-0.5 cun
			Urinary stones	0.3-0.5 cun
			Uterine tumor	0.3-0.5 cun
			Vaginitis	0.3-0.5 cun

Notes:

Tung Acupuncture: A Quick Reference Guide

Point	Name Pinyin	English Name	Indications	Insertion
66.04	Hou Zhu	Fire Master	Allergy, nasal	0.3-0.8 cun
			Angina pectoris	0.3-0.8 cun
			Bone diseases	0.3-0.8 cun
			Bone swelling	0.3-0.8 cun
			Breech presentation (At childbirth)	0.3-0.8 cun
			Cardiac arrest	0.3-0.8 cun
			Cardiac diseases	0.3-0.8 cun
			Coma	0.3-0.8 cun
			Difficult delivery	0.3-0.8 cun
			Dysuria	0.3-0.8 cun
			Feet pain	0.3-0.8 cun
			Glaucoma	0.3-0.8 cun
			Hand pain	0.3-0.8 cun
			Hand pain (Flexor tendonitis, palm side)	0.3-0.8 cun
			Headache	0.3-0.8 cun
			Headache d/t Heart disease	0.3-0.8 cun
			Heart paralysis (For resuscitation)	0.3-0.8 cun
			Joint pain	0.3-0.8 cun
			Liver disease	0.3-0.8 cun
			Metritis (Uterine inflammation)	0.3-0.8 cun
			Nasal bleeding	0.3-0.8 cun
			Nervousness	0.3-0.8 cun
			Pain in hands and feet	0.3-0.8 cun
			Peptic ulcer	0.3-0.8 cun
			Pudendum swelling	0.3-0.8 cun
			Stomach disease	0.3-0.8 cun
			Tendon diseases	0.3-0.8 cun
			Urinary stones	0.3-0.8 cun
			Uterine tumor	0.3-0.8 cun
			Vaginitis	0.3-0.8 cun

Notes:

110

Point	Name Pinyin	English Name	Indications	Insertion
66.05	Men Jin	Door Gold	Abdominal pain	0.5 cun
			Abdominal pain & distension (Upper)	0.5 cun
			Abdominal pain lateral lower	0.5 cun
			Appendicitis	0.5 cun
			Chest pain lateral	0.5 cun
			Cholecystitis	0.5 cun
			Common cold	0.5 cun
			Diarrhea acute (Imodium point)	0.5 cun
			Diarrhea acute/chronic	0.5 cun
			Dysentery	0.5 cun
			Dysmenorrhea	0.5 cun
			Enteritis	0.5 cun
			Enteritis acute	0.5 cun
			Enteritis chronic	0.5 cun
			Eyes, difficulty opening	0.5 cun
			Gastritis	0.5 cun
			Headache: Migraines pain at Taiyang (Also Yangming)	0.5 cun
			Large intestine diseases	0.5 cun
			Large intestine distending pain	0.5 cun
			Liver stagnation	0.5 cun
			Mandible pain (Difficulty opening mouth)	0.5 cun
			Migraine	Micro-puncture
			Mouth (Difficulty opening) mandible pain	0.5 cun
			Nasal obstruction	0.5 cun
			Poor appetite	0.5 cun
			Ptosis of the eyes Due to myasthenia	0.5 cun
			Stomach diseases	0.5 cun
			Stomach distension	0.5 cun
			Urticaria	0.5 cun
66.06	Mu Liu	Wood Stay	Aplastic anemia	0.3-0.5 cun
			Cholecystitis	0.3-0.5 cun
			Cirhossis	1.5-2.5 cun
			Erythropenia	0.3-0.5 cun
			Fatigue	0.3-0.5 cun
			Finger numbness	0.3-0.5 cun
			Finger pain	0.3-0.5 cun
			Gall bladder disease	0.3-0.5 cun
			Hyper-Leucocytosis	0.3-0.5 cun
			Indigestion	0.3-0.5 cun
			Leucopenia	0.3-0.5 cun
			Leukemia	0.3-0.5 cun
			Liver disease	0.3-0.5 cun
			Liver disease, chronic	0.3-0.5 cun
			Liver disharmony	0.3-0.5 cun
			Middle finger (Can't bend)	0.3-0.5 cun
			Poliomyelitis	0.3-0.5 cun
			Spleen disharmony	0.3-0.5 cun
			Splenomegaly	0.3-0.5 cun

Tung Acupuncture: A Quick Reference Guide

Point	Name Pinyin	English Name	Indications	Insertion
66.07	Mu Dou	Wood Scoop	Aplastic anemia	0.3-0.5 cun
			Cholecystitis (GB inflammation)	0.3-0.5 cun
			Cirhossis	1.5-2.5 cun
			Erythropenia	0.3-0.5 cun
			Fatigue	0.3-0.5 cun
			Finger numbness	0.3-0.5 cun
			Hyper-Leucocytosis	0.3-0.5 cun
			Indigestion	0.3-0.5 cun
			Leucopenia	0.3-0.5 cun
			Liver disease	0.3-0.5 cun
			Liver disharmony	0.3-0.5 cun
			Poliomyelitis	0.3-0.5 cun
			Spleen disharmony	0.3-0.5 cun
			Splenomegaly	0.3-0.5 cun
66.08	Liu Wan	Sixth Finish	Arm pain (Upper)	0.3-0.5 cun
			Hemorrhagic disorders	0.3-0.5 cun
			Migraine	0.3-0.5 cun
			Nasal bleeding	0.3-0.5 cun
66.09	Shui Qu	Water Curve	Abdominal swelling (Due to flatulence)	0.5-1.0 cun
			Arthralgia	0.5-1.0 cun
			Cervical neuralgia	0.5-1.0 cun
			Clavicle pain (Frontal)	0.5-1.0 cun
			Edema peripheral	0.5-1.0 cun
			Flatulence (Abdominal swelling)	0.5-1.0 cun
			Headache: Migraines	0.5-1.0 cun
			Indigestion	0.5-1.0 cun
			Limbs atrophy (muscle wasting)	0.5-1.0 cun
			Lumbago	0.5-1.0 cun
			Peripheral edema	0.5-1.0 cun
66.10	Huo Lian	Fire Connection	Dizziness (Due to HTN)	0.5-0.8 cun
			Fatigue	0.5-0.8 cun
			Heart weakness Due to Hypertension.	0.5-0.8 cun
			Limbs weakness	0.5-0.8 cun
			Middle age house wife syndrome	0.5-0.8 cun
			Palpitations	0.5-0.8 cun
			Vertigo	0.5-0.8 cun

Notes:

112

Tung Acupuncture: A Quick Reference Guide

Point	Name Pinyin	English Name	Indications	Insertion
66.11	Hou Ju	Fire Chrysanthemum	Abdominal pain lateral lower	0.5-0.8 cun
			Blurred vision	0.5-0.8 cun
			Dizziness (Due to HTN)	0.5-0.8 cun
			Eye soreness	0.5-0.8 cun
			Eyelid edema	0.5-0.8 cun
			Finger numbness	0.5-0.8 cun
			Foot pain	0.5-0.8 cun
			Fullness in head	0.5-0.8 cun
			Hand numbness	0.5-0.8 cun
			Headache: Frontal	0.5-0.8 cun
			Hypertension	0.5-0.8 cun
			Neck movement restriction	0.5-0.8 cun
			Numbness of hand	0.5-0.8 cun
			Palpitations	0.5-0.8 cun
			Ptosis of the eyes Due to myasthenia	0.5-0.8 cun
			Restriction of neck movement	0.5-0.8 cun
			Vertigo	0.5-0.8 cun
			Vision debility	0.5-0.8 cun
66.12	Huo San	Fire Scatter	Back (Low) soreness	0.5-1.0 cun
			Back pain	0.5-1.0 cun
			Blurred vision	0.5-0.8 cun
			Conjunctivitis	0.5-1.0 cun
			Dizziness (Due to HTN)	0.5-1.0 cun
			Headache	0.5-1.0 cun
			Headache (tension)	0.5-1.0 cun
			Kidney Deficiency	0.5-1.0 cun
			Low back pain	0.5-1.0 cun
			Meningitis (Rigidity of neck)	0.5-1.0 cun
			Vision debility	0.5-1.0 cun
66.13	Shui Jing	Water Crystal	Fibroids	0.5-1.0 cun
			Metritis	0.5-1.0 cun
			Pelvic congestion syndrome	0.5-1.0 cun
			Pelvic infloamatory disease	0.5-1.0 cun
			Pelvic pain	0.5-1.0 cun
			Uterine myoma	0.5-1.0 cun
66.14	Shui Xiang	Water Phase	Back pain low	0.3-0.5 cun
			Cataract	0.3-0.5 cun
			Chest pain to abdomen along Ren.	0.3-0.5 cun
			Nephritis	0.3-0.5 cun
			Preeclampsia	0.3-0.5 cun
			Spinal pain	0.3-0.5 cun
66.15	Shui Xian	Water Fairy	Back pain low	0.5 cun
			Cataract	0.5 cun
			Nephritis	0.5 cun
			Preeclampsia	0.5 cun
			Spinal pain	0.5 cun
66.16	Da Zhong	Large Bell	Wrist pain (Carple tunnel, arthritis and the like)	1.0-1.5 cun

Point	Name Pinyin	English Name	Indications	Insertion
77.01	Zheng Jin	Upright Tendon	Back pain low	0.5-0.8 cun
			Brain tumor	0.5-0.8 cun
			Cramp of the foot	0.5-0.8 cun
			Cranial bone Enlargement	0.5-0.8 cun
			Foot cramp	0.5-0.8 cun
			Headache: Occipital	0.5-0.8 cun
			Hydrocephalus	0.5-0.8 cun
			Lumbago	0.5-0.8 cun
			Neck pain (All types)	0.5-0.8 cun
			Neck pain (Due to herniated cervical disc and S/S)	0.5–0.8 cun
			Neck pain (Herniated discs) Cervical discs C1-C7.	0.5-0.8 cun
			Occiput pain	0.5-0.8 cun
			Spinal pain	0.5-0.8 cun
			Spinal pain (Neck)	0.5-0.8 cun
			Spinal sprain acute	0.5-0.8 cun
77.02	Zheng Zong	Uprightness Ancestry	Neck pain (Due to herniated cervical disc and S/S)	0.5-0.8 cun
			Back pain low	0.5-0.8 cun
			Headache: Occipital	0.5-0.8 cun
			Hydrocephalus	0.5-0.8 cun
			Lumbago	0.5-0.8 cun
			Neck pain (All types)	0.5-0.8 cun
			Occiput pain	0.5-0.8 cun
			Spinal pain	0.5-0.8 cun
			Spinal pain (Neck)	0.5-0.8 cun
77.03	Zheng Shi	Upright Scholar	Back ache (Bilateral)	0.5-1.0 cun
			Lumbago	0.5-1.0 cun
			Sciatica	0.5-1.0 cun
			Shoulder-hand syndrome (Mainly pain)	0.5-1.0 cun
			Spinal pain	0.5-1.0 cun
77.04	Bo Qiu	Catching Ball	Back ache (Bilateral)	1.0-2.0 cun
			Cholera with convulsions	1.0-2.0 cun
			Cramp, leg	1.0-2.0 cun
			Enterogastritis with convulsions	1.0-2.0 cun
			Epistaxis	1.0-2.0 cun
			Gastro-enteritis	1.0-2.0 cun
			Leg cramp	1.0-2.0 cun
			Lumbago	1.0-2.0 cun
			Scapular pain	1.0-2.0 cun
			Spinal sprain acute	1.0-2.0 cun

Notes:

114

Point	Name Pinyin	English Name	Indications	Insertion
77.05	Yi Zhong	First Weight	Breast augmentation	1.0-2.0 cun
			Breast tumors	1.0-2.0 cun
			Cosmetic	1.0-2.0 cun
			Costalgia (Right side in females)	1.0-2.0 cun
			Facial nerve palsy	1.0-2.0 cun
			Hyper thyroidism	1.0-2.0 cun
			Intraductal papillomas	1.0-2.0 cun
			Liver cirrhosis	1.0-2.0 cun
			Mastitis	1.0-2.0 cun
			Meningitis	1.0-2.0 cun
			Rib pain	1.0-2.0 cun
			Splenomegaly	1.0-2.0 cun
			Tonsillitis	1.0-2.0 cun
77.06	Er Zhong	Second Weight	Breast augmentation	1.0-2.0 cun
			Breast tumors	1.0-2.0 cun
			Costalgia (Right side in females)	1.0-2.0 cun
			Facial nerve palsy	1.0-2.0 cun
			Hyper thyroidism	1.0-2.0 cun
			Intraductal papillomas	1.0-2.0 cun
			Liver cirrhosis	1.0-2.0 cun
			Mastitis	1.0-2.0 cun
			Meningitis	1.0-2.0 cun
			Rib pain	1.0-2.0 cun
			Splenomegaly	1.0-2.0 cun
			Tonsillitis	1.0-2.0 cun
77.07	San Zhong	Third Weight	Brain tumor	1.0-2.0 cun
			Breast augmentation	1.0-2.0 cun
			Breast tumors	1.0-2.0 cun
			Costalgia (Right side in females)	1.0-2.0 cun
			Earache	1.0-2.0 cun
			Facial nerve palsy	1.0-2.0 cun
			Facial numbness	1.0-2.0 cun
			Facial paralysis	1.0-2.0 cun
			Headache: Migraines	1.0-2.0 cun
			Hyper thyroidism	1.0-2.0 cun
			Intraductal papillomas	1.0-2.0 cun
			Lacrimation in wind	1.0-2.0 cun
			Liver cirrhosis	1.0-2.0 cun
			Mastitis	1.0-2.0 cun
			Meningitis	1.0-2.0 cun
			Rib pain	1.0-2.0 cun
			Splenomegaly	Micro-puncture
			Tonsillitis	1.0-2.0 cun
			Vertigo severe case	1.0-2.0 cun
			Zygomatic pain	Micro-puncture

115

Tung Acupuncture: A Quick Reference Guide

Point	Name Pinyin	English Name	Indications	Insertion
77.08	Si Hua Shang	4 Upper Flowers	Asthma	2.0-3.0 cun
			Coronary artery disease	3.0-3.5 cun
			Dizziness	3.0-3.5 cun
			Dysuria	2.0-3.0 cun
			Dysuria due to prostatitis	2.0-3.0 cun
			Edema of the leg	3.0-3.5 cun
			Frozen shoulder	2.0-3.0 cun
			Gastritis	Micro-puncture
			Oral ulceration	2.0-3.0 cun
			Palpitations	3.0-3.5 cun
			Poor appetite	2.0-3.0 cun
			Prostatitis	2.0-3.0 cun
			Shoulder difficlty lifting	2.0-3.0 cun
			Stomach ache (Acute)	2.0-3.0 cun
			Stomach diseases	Micro-puncture
			Toothache	3.0-3.5 cun
			Vomiting	3.0-3.5 cun
77.09	Si Hua Z7hong	4 Middle Flowers	Abdominal pain lower	Micro-puncture
			Acute stomachache	Micro-puncture
			Adhesive capsulitis	Micro-puncture
			Appendicitis	Micro-puncture
			Arm pain (Upper)	Micro-puncture
			Arteriosclerosis	Micro-puncture
			Asthma	2.0-3.0 cun
			Asthmatic breathing	Micro-puncture
			Athrosclerosis	Micro-puncture
			Bone swelling	Micro-puncture
			Cardiac arrest	Micro-puncture
			Cardiac pain	Micro-puncture
			Carditis	Micro-puncture
			Chest injury (Impact trauma)	Micro-puncture
			Chest oppression	Micro-puncture
			Chest stuffiness	Micro-puncture
			Cholera with convulsions	2.0-3.0 cun
			Cirhossis	Micro-puncture
			Colic abdominal pain	Micro-puncture
			Diarrhea acute	Micro-puncture
			Diarrhea severe	Micro-puncture
			Elbow joint pain	Micro-puncture
			Emphysema	Micro-puncture
			Enteritis acute	Micro-puncture
			Enterogastritis with convulsions	Micro-puncture
			Finger pain	Micro-puncture
			Finger pain index finger	Micro-puncture
			Frozen shoulder	2.0-3.0 cun
			Headache: Frontal	Micro-puncture
			Heart disease severe	Micro-puncture
			Heel pain	Micro-puncture
			Heel spurs	Micro-puncture
			Hypertension	Micro-puncture
			Internal organ disease	Micro-puncture

Point	Name Pinyin	English Name	Indications	Insertion
77.09	Si Hua Zhong	4 Middle Flowers	Knee joint pain	Micro-puncture
			Knee spurs	Micro-puncture
			Liver GB diseases	Micro-puncture
			Myocardial infarction	2.0-3.0 cun
			Myocarditis	Micro-puncture
			Ophthalmalgia	Micro-puncture
			Oral ulceration	2.0-3.0 cun
			Pain in the heel	Micro-puncture
			Pleurisy	Micro-puncture
			Pleuritis	Micro-puncture
			Regurgitation	Micro-puncture
			Restless	Micro-puncture
			Sciatica Due to bone spurs	Micro-puncture
			Shoulder difficlty lifting	Micro-puncture
			Spinal vertebra tenderness	Micro-puncture
			Spinal vertebrae spur	Micro-puncture
			Spur of the knee	Micro-puncture
			Spurs	Micro-puncture
			Stomach ache (Acute)	Micro-puncture
			Stomach diseases	Micro-puncture
			Stomach ulceration	Micro-puncture
			Stomachache	Micro-puncture
			Tachycardia	Micro-puncture
			Teburculosis	Micro-puncture
			T-M joint pain	2.0-3.0 cun
			Ulcertation of the Duodenum	Micro-puncture
			Vomiting	Micro-puncture
77.10	Si Hua Fu	4 Append Flowers	Adhesive capsulitis	Micro-puncture
			Arteriosclerosis	Micro-puncture
			Asthma	Micro-punture
			Bone swelling	Micro-puncture
			Carditis	Micro-puncture
			Disc problems (Severe case)	Micro-puncture
			Elbow pain, inner (little league pitcher's elbow)	Micro-puncture
			Emphysema	Micro-puncture
			Enteritis	Micro-puncture
			Frozen shoulder	Micro-puncture
			Golfers elbow	Micro-puncture
			Ophthalmalgia	Micro-puncture
			Spinal vertebra tenderness	Micro-puncture
			Spinal vertebrae spur	Micro-puncture
			Spurs	Micro-puncture
			Stomachache	Micro-puncture

Point	Name Pinyin	English Name	Indications	Insertion
77.11	Si Hua Xia	4 Lower Flowers	Bruxism	0.5-1.0 cun
			Disc problems (Severe case)	0.5-1.0 cun
			Dyspnoea	0.5-1.0 cun
			Edema peripheral	0.5-1.0 cun
			Enteritis	0.5-1.0 cun
			Heel pain	0.5-1.0 cun
			Heel spurs	0.5-1.0 cun
			Knee joint pain	0.5-1.0 cun
			Knee spurs	0.5-1.0 cun
			Pain in the heel	0.5-1.0 cun
			Sciatica Due to bone spurs	0.5-1.0 cun
			Stomachache	0.5-1.0 cun
			Teeth clenching at night Bruxism	0.5-1.0 cun
77.12	Fu Chang	Bowels Intestine	Bruxism	0.5-1.0 cun
			Disc problems (Severe case)	0.5-1.0 cun
			Dyspnoea	0.5-1.0 cun
			Edema peripheral	0.5-1.0 cun
			Enteritis	0.5-1.0 cun
			Stomachache	0.5-1.0 cun
			Teeth clenching at night Bruxism	0.5-1.0 cun
77.13	Si Hua Li	4 Inner Flowers	Coronary artery disease	1.5-2.0 cun
			Enterogastritis	1.5-2.0 cun
			Frozen shoulder	1.5-2.0 cun
			Palpitations	1.5-2.0 cun
			Vomiting	1.5-2.0 cun

Notes:

Point	Name Pinyin	English Name	Indications	Insertion
77.14	Si Hua Wai	4 Lateral Flowers	Abdominal pain lower	Micro-puncture
			Acute enteritis	1.0-1.5 cun
			Appendicitis	1.0-1.5 cun
			Asthma	1.0-1.5 cun
			Asthmatic breathing	Micro-puncture
			Athrosclerosis	Micro-puncture
			Cardiac pain	1.0-1.5 cun
			Chest injury (Impact trauma)	1.0-1.5 cun
			Chest oppression	Micro-puncture
			Chest stuffiness	Micro-puncture
			Cholera with convulsions	1.0-1.5 cun
			Chronic sinusitis	1.0-1.5 cun
			Colic abdominal pain	Micro-puncture
			Diarrhea acute	Micro-puncture
			Diarrhea severe	Micro-puncture
			Ear infection	1.0-1.5 cun
			Ear pain	1.0-1.5 cun
			Earache	1.0-1.5 cun
			Elbow pain (Lateral Humeral epicondylitis)	1.0-1.5 cun
			Emphysema	1.0-1.5 cun
			Enteritis acute	1.0-1.5 cun
			Enterogastritis with convulsions	Micro-puncture
			Facial palsy	1.0-1.5 cun
			Facial paralysis	1.0-1.5 cun
			Frozen shoulder	1.0-1.5 cun
			Headache	1.0-1.5 cun
			Headache: Migraines	1.0-1.5 cun
			Heart disease severe	1.0-1.5 cun
			Hypertension	1.0-1.5 cun
			Intercostal neuralgia (Shingles etc..)	1.0-1.5 cun
			Internal organ disease	0.5-1.0 cun
			Lateral epicondylitis	1.0-1.5 cun
			Liver GB diseases	Micro-puncture
			Migraine	1.0-1.5 cun
			Myocardial infarction	1.0-1.5 cun
			Myocarditis	0.5-1.0 cun
			Obesity	Micro-puncture
			Otitis media Chronic in children	Micro-puncture
			Scapular pain	1.0-1.5 cun
			Sciatica Along GB Meridian	Micro-puncture
			Shoulder/arm pain,	1.0-1.5 cun
			Stomach diseases	0.5-1.0 cun
			Stomach ulceration	0.5-1.0 cun
			Tachycardia	0.5-1.0 cun
			Teburculosis	Micro-puncture
			Tennis elbow	1.0-1.5 cun
			Toothache	1.0-1.5 cun
			Ulcertation of the Duodenum	Micro-puncture

Point	Name Pinyin	English Name	Indications	Insertion
77.15	Shang Chun	Upper Lip	Aphthae (Mouth ulcer)	Micro-puncture
			Cold sore	Micro-puncture
			Lip tenderness	Micro-puncture
			Mouth ulcer	Micro-puncture
			Oral ulceration	Micro-puncture
77.16	Xia Chun	Lower Lip	Aphthae (Mouth ulcer)	Micro-puncture
			Cold sore	Micro-puncture
			Lip tenderness	Micro-puncture
			Oral ulceration	Micro-puncture
77.17	Tian Huang	Heaven Emperor	Acid reflux	0.5-1.0 cun
			Arthritis rheumatoid	0.5-1.0 cun
			Diabetes mellitus	0.5-1.0 cun
			Dysuria	0.5-1.0 cun
			Dysuria due to prostatitis	0.5-1.0 cun
			Edema of the leg	0.5-1.0 cun
			Esophageal reflux	0.5-1.0 cun
			Excessive stomach acid	0.5-1.0 cun
			Gastric acid excessive	0.5-1.0 cun
			Gastric reflux excessive	0.5-1.0 cun
			Glomerulonephritis (Pitting edema)	0.5-1.0 cun
			Headache: Frontal	0.5-1.0 cun
			Hypertension	0.5-1.0 cun
			Insomnia	0.5-1.0 cun
			Prostatitis	0.5-1.0 cun
			Regurgitation	0.5-1.0 cun
			Urticaria	Micro-puncture
77.18	Shen Guan	Kidney Gate	Acid reflux	1.5-2.0 cun
			Albuminuria	1.5-2.0 cun
			Anemia	1.5-2.0 cun
			Astigmatism	1.5-2.0 cun
			Balanitis	1.5-2.0 cun
			Blurred vision	1.5-2.0 cun
			Bronchitis (Chronic)	1.5-2.0 cun
			Cataract	1.5-2.0 cun
			Chest & back pain	1.5-2.0 cun
			Cloudiness thinking and fatigue (Neurasthenia)	1.5-2.0 cun
			Diabetes mellitus	1.5-2.0 cun
			Dysuria	1.5-2.0 cun
			Edema of the limbs	1.5-2.0 cun
			Elbow pain (Lateral Humeral epicondylitis)	1.5-2.0 cun
			Epilepsy, idiopathic	1.5-2.0 cun
			Essential tremor	1.5-2.0 cun
			Excessive stomach acid	1.5-2.0 cun
			Eye dark rings	1.5-2.0 cun
			Eye twitching	1.5-2.0 cun
			Eyeball deviation	1.5-2.0 cun
			Eyelid bags	1.5-2.0 cun
			Finger numbness	1.5-2.0 cun

Tung Acupuncture: A Quick Reference Guide

Point	Name Pinyin	English Name	Indications	Insertion
77.18	Shen Guan	Kidney Gate	Frequent urination	1.5-2.0 cun
			Frozen shoulder	1.5-2.0 cun
			Galacturia	1.5-2.0 cun
			Glaucoma	1.5-2.0 cun
			Hand pain difficulty holding object	1.5-2.0 cun
			Headache	1.5-2.0 cun
			Headache Taiyang	1.5-2.0 cun
			Headache: Frontal	1.5-2.0 cun
			Hematuria	1.5-2.0 cun
			Hemiplegia	1.5-2.0 cun
			Hemiplegia due to K deficiency	1.5-2.0 cun
			Hyper-Leucocytosis	1.5-2.0 cun
			Hypertension renal	1.5-2.0 cun
			Hysteria	1.5-2.0 cun
			Insomnia	1.5-2.0 cun
			Intentional tremor	1.5-2.0 cun
			Joint pain Shoulder	1.5-2.0 cun
			Kidney deficiency	1.5-2.0 cun
			Lacrimation due to wind exposure	1.5-2.0 cun
			Leg numbness	1.5-2.0 cun
			Lower back pain	1.5-2.0 cun
			Lower back pain due to Kidney deficiency	1.5-2.0 cun
			Multiple sclerosis	1.5-2.0 cun
			Myiodesopsia	1.5-2.0 cun
			Optic atrophy	1.5-2.0 cun
			Parkinson's disease	1.5-2.0 cun
			Premature ejaculation	1.5-2.0 cun
			Regurgitation	1.5-2.0 cun
			Renal disorders	1.5-2.0 cun
			Seminal emissions	1.5-2.0 cun
			Shen-K'uei syndrome	1.5-2.0 cun
			Shingles	1.5-2.0 cun
			Shoulder & back pain	1.5-2.0 cun
			Shoulder difficlty lifting	1.5-2.0 cun
			Shoulder joint pain	1.5-2.0 cun
			Squint	1.5-2.0 cun
			Strabismus (Squint)	1.5-2.0 cun
			Tennis Elbow	1.5-2.0 cun
			Toe numbness	1.5-2.0 cun
			Twitching of the eye	1.5-2.0 cun
			Urination difficulty	1.5-2.0 cun
			Urination frequent	1.5-2.0 cun
			Vertigo	1.5-2.0 cun
			Vertigo due to pathological changes of cerebral nerves.	1.5-2.0 cun
			Vision blurred	1.5-2.0 cun

Notes:

Auto immune

121

Tung Acupuncture: A Quick Reference Guide

Point	Name Pinyin	English Name	Indications	Insertion
77.19	Di Huang	Earthly Emperor	Balanitis	1.0-1.5 cun
			Cataract	1.0-1.5 cun
			Cloudiness thinking and fatigue (Neurasthenia)	1.0-1.5 cun
			Diabetes mellitus	1.0-1.5 cun
			Dysuria	1.0-1.5 cun
			Edema	1.0-1.5 cun
			Edema of the limbs	1.0-1.5 cun
			Eyeball deviation	1.0-1.5 cun
			Fibroids (Uterine myoma)	1.0-1.5 cun
			Galacturia	1.0-1.5 cun
			Glaucoma	1.0-1.5 cun
			Glomerulonephritis (Pitting edema)	1.0-1.5 cun
			Gonorrhea	1.0-1.5 cun
			Haematurea	1.0-1.5 cun
			Hyper-Leucocytosis	1.0-1.5 cun
			Impotence	1.0-1.5 cun
			Impotence & Premature ejaculation	1.0-1.5 cun
			Insomnia	1.0-1.5 cun
			Lacrimation due to wind exposure	1.0-1.5 cun
			Leg numbness	1.0-1.5 cun
			Lower back pain	1.0-1.5 cun
			Parkinson's disease	1.0-1.5 cun
			Premature ejaculation	1.0-1.5 cun
			Renal disorders	1.0-1.5 cun
			Seminal emissions	1.0-1.5 cun
			Toe numbness	1.0-1.5 cun
			Uterine myoma (Fibroids)	1.0-1.5 cun
			Vertigo due to pathological changes of cerebral nerves.	1.0-1.5 cun
77.20	Si Zhi	Four Limbs	Alcoholic neuritis (Pain in the hands & feet)	1.0-1.5 cun
			Diabetes mellitus	1.0-1.5 cun
			Hip pain	1.0-1.5 cun
			Neck pain	1.0-1.5 cun

Notes:

122

© Theodore L. Zombolas PhD (AM), LAc, Dipl.Ac. (NCCAOM). ©

Point	Name Pinyin	English Name	Indications	Insertion
77.21	Ren Huang	Man Emperor	Balanitis	0.6-1.2 cun
			Cataract	0.6-1.2 cun
			Cloudiness thinking and fatigue (Neurasthenia)	0.6-1.2 cun
			Diabetes mellitus	0.6-1.2 cun
			Dizziness	0.6-1.2 cun
			Dysuria	0.6-1.2 cun
			Early ejaculation	0.6-1.2 cun
			Edema of the limbs	0.6-1.2 cun
			Eyeball deviation	0.6-1.2 cun
			Eyes, difficulty opening	0.6-1.2 cun
			Galacturia	0.6-1.2 cun
			Glaucoma	0.6-1.2 cun
			Gonorrhea	0.6-1.2 cun
			Hands numbness Due to Diabetes	0.6-1.2 cun
			Hematuria	0.6-1.2 cun
			Hyper-Leucocytosis	0.6-1.2 cun
			Impotence	0.6-1.2 cun
			Insomnia	0.6-1.2 cun
			Lacrimation due to wind exposure	0.6-1.2 cun
			Leg numbness	0.6-1.2 cun
			Low back pain	0.6-1.2 cun
			Lumbago	0.6-1.2 cun
			Neck pain (Acute)	0.6-1.2 cun
			Parkinson's disease	0.6-1.2 cun
			Premature ejaculation	0.6-1.2 cun
			Renal disorders	0.6-1.2 cun
			Seminal emissions	0.6-1.2 cun
			Toe numbness	0.6-1.2 cun
			Ulnar neuritis (Numbness & tingling)	0.6-1.2 cun
			Urticaria	Micro-puncture
			Vertigo due to pathological changes of cerebral nerves.	0.6-1.2 cun

Notes:

123

Point	Name Pinyin	English Name	Indications	Insertion
77.22	Ce San Li	Lateral 3 Mile	Arm pain (Upper)	0.5-1.0 cun
			Common cold	0.5-1.0 cun
			Earache	0.5-1.0 cun
			Eye twitching	0.5-1.0 cun
			Facial nerve palsy	0.5-1.0 cun
			Facial numbness	0.5-1.0 cun
			Facial paralysis	0.5-1.0 cun
			Facial paralysis Chronic cases	0.5-1.0 cun
			Facial paralysis Unilateral	0.5-1.0 cun
			Facial spasm	0.5-1.0 cun
			Gingivitis	0.5-1.0 cun
			Hand numbness	0.5-1.0 cun
			Hand pain difficulty holding object	0.5-1.0 cun
			Hand sorness	0.5-1.0 cun
			Headache	0.5-1.0 cun
			Headache (Temporal, tension)	0.5-1.0 cun
			Headache, Yangming & Shaoyang	0.5-1.0 cun
			Headache: Migraines, disorders of Yangming and/or Shaoyang	0.5-1.0 cun
			Nasal obstruction	0.5-1.0 cun
			Otitis media	Micro-puncture
			Pain of the wrist joint	0.5-1.0 cun
			Soreness of the hand	0.5-1.0 cun
			Sublingual swelling	0.5-1.0 cun
			Tenosynovitis	0.5-1.0 cun
			Toothache	0.5-1.0 cun
			Twitching of the eye	0.5-1.0 cun
			Wrist joint pain	0.5-1.0 cun
			Zygomatic pain	0.5-1.0 cun

Notes:

Point	Name Pinyin	English Name	Indications	Insertion
77.23	Ce Xia San Li	Below Lateral 3 Mile	Acromion pain	0.5-1.0 cun
			Earache	0.5-1.0 cun
			Eye twitching	0.5-1.0 cun
			Facial nerve palsy	0.5-1.0 cun
			Facial numbness	0.5-1.0 cun
			Facial paralysis	0.5-1.0 cun
			Facial paralysis Chronic cases	0.5-1.0 cun
			Facial spasm	0.5-1.0 cun
			Gingivitis	0.5-1.0 cun
			Hand numbness	0.5-1.0 cun
			Hand pain difficulty holding object	0.5-1.0 cun
			Hand sorness	0.5-1.0 cun
			Headache	0.5-1.0 cun
			Headache, Yangming & Shaoyang	0.5-1.0 cun
			Headache: Migraines, disorders of Yangming and/or Shaoyang	0.5-1.0 cun
			Otitis media	0.5-1.0 cun
			Pain of the acromion	0.5-1.0 cun
			Pain of the wrist joint	0.5-1.0 cun
			Soreness of the hand	0.5-1.0 cun
			Sublingual swelling	0.5-1.0 cun
			Toothache	0.5-1.0 cun
			Twitching of the eye	0.5-1.0 cun
			Wrist joint pain	0.5-1.0 cun
			Zygomatic pain	0.5-1.0 cun
77.24	Zu Qian Jin	Foot 1000 Gold	Enteritis acute	0.5-1.0 cun
			Enteritis chronic	0.5-1.0 cun
			Frozen shoulder	0.5-1.0 cun
			Large intestine diseases	0.5-1.0 cun
			Laryngitis	0.5-1.0 cun
			Lung diseases	0.5-1.0 cun
			Peritonsillar abscess	0.5-1.0 cun
			Quinsy	0.5-1.0 cun
			Shoulder difficlty lifting	0.5-1.0 cun
			Sore throat	0.5-1.0 cun
			Supraspinatus tendonitis	0.5-1.0 cun
			Thyroiditis	0.5-1.0 cun
			Tonsillitis	0.5-1.0 cun
77.25	Zu Wu Jin	Foot 5 Gold	Enteritis acute	0.5-1.0 cun
			Frozen shoulder	0.5-1.0 cun
			Large intestine diseases	0.5-1.0 cun
			Laryngitis	0.5-1.0 cun
			Lung diseases	0.5-1.0 cun
			Peritonsillar abscess	0.5-1.0 cun
			Quinsy	0.5-1.0 cun
			Shoulder difficlty lifting	0.5-1.0 cun
			Sore throat	0.5-1.0 cun
			Supraspinatus tendonitis	0.5-1.0 cun
			Thyroiditis	0.5-1.0 cun
			Tonsillitis	0.5-1.0 cun

Tung Acupuncture: A Quick Reference Guide

Point	Name Pinyin	English Name	Indications	Insertion
77.26	Qi Hu	Seven Tigers	Chest pain	0.5-0.8 cun
			Clavicle pain (Frontal)	0.5-0.8 cun
			Clavicular pain	0.5-0.8 cun
			Fractures	0.5-0.8 cun
			Impact trauma	0.5-0.8 cun
			Joint sublixation	0.5-0.8 cun
			Pleuritis (Pneumonia or infectious disease)	0.5-0.8 cun
			Rib pain	0.5-0.8 cun
			Scapulalgia	0.5-0.8 cun
			Sternum pain	0.5-0.8 cun
			Trauma (Impact)	0.5-0.8 cun
77.27	Wai San Guan	Outer 3 Gates	Abscess	1.0-1.5 cun.
			Breast augmentation	1.0-1.5 cun.
			Breast cancer	1.0-1.5 cun.
			Breast fibroadenomas (Benign tumor)	1.0-1.5 cun.
			Infections parotitis (mumps)	1.0-1.5 cun.
			Laryngitis	1.0-1.5 cun.
			Mumps	1.0-1.5 cun.
			Obesity	Micro-puncture
			Shoulder frozen	1.0-1.5 cun.
			Shoulder pain syndrome (Any pain from shoulder to wrist & scapula)	1.0-1.5 cun
			Tonsillitis	1.0-1.5 cun.
77.28	Guang Ming	Bright Light	Shingles	0.5-1.0 cun
			Astigmatism	0.5-1.0 cun
			Blurred vision	0.5-1.0 cun
			Myiodesopsia	0.5-1.0 cun
			Optic atrophy	0.5-1.0 cun
			Vision blurred	0.5-1.0 cun
			Eyes, difficulty opening	0.5-1.0 cun
			Astigmatism (Distorted vision)	0.5-1.0 cun
			Cataract	0.5-1.0 cun
			Diplopia (Double vision)	0.5-1.0 cun
			Double vision	0.5-1.0 cun
			Drooping of eye lid (Ptosis)	0.5-1.0 cun
			Eye dryness	0.5-1.0 cun
			Eye pain (Burning, tearing, eye strain)	0.5-1.0 cun
			Ptosis	0.5-1.0 cun
77.29	Nei Xi Yan	Medial Eye of The Knee	Liver cirrhosis	1.0-1.5 cun

Notes:

126

Point	Name Pinyin	English Name	Indications	Insertion
88.01	Tong Guan	Penetrating Gate	Acute Cardiac rheumatism	0.3-0.5 cun
			Angina pectoris	0.3-0.5 cun
			Bradicardia	0.3-0.5 cun
			Cardiac pain	0.3-0.5 cun
			Cerebral ischemia	0.3-0.5 cun
			Chest pain	0.3-0.5 cun
			Coronary artery disease	0.3-0.5 cun
			Dizziness	0.3-0.5 cun
			Erysipelas (Skin infection)	0.3-0.5 cun
			Extremities pain	0.3-0.5 cun
			Floating vision	0.3-0.5 cun
			Gastritis	0.3-0.5 cun
			Heart disease	0.3-0.5 cun
			Heart issues	0.3-0.5 cun
			Hypertension	0.3-0.5 cun
			Middle finger numbness	0.3-0.5 cun
			Myocardial infarction	0.3-0.5 cun
			Myocarditis	0.3-0.5 cun
			Nasal disease	0.3-0.5 cun
			Palpitations	0.3-0.5 cun
			Paraesthesia	0.3-0.5 cun
			Pericarditis	0.3-0.5 cun
			Rheumatic fever (Esp. arthritis)	0.3-0.5 cun
			Skin infection (Erysipelas)	0.3-0.5 cun
			Stomach diseases	0.3-0.5 cun
			Stomach distension	0.3-0.5 cun
			Stomachache	0.3-0.5 cun
			TIA	0.3-0.5 cun
			Vertigo due to anemia	0.3-0.5 cun
			Vertigo: due to cerebral anemia	0.3-0.5 cun

Notes:

Point	Name Pinyin	English Name	Indications	Insertion
88.02	Tong Shan	Passing Mountain	Acute Cardiac rheumatism	0.5-0.8 cun
			Angina pectoris	0.5-0.8 cun
			Bradicardia	0.5-0.8 cun
			Cardiac pain	0.5-0.8 cun
			Cerebral ischemia	0.5-0.8 cun
			Chest pain	0.5-0.8 cun
			Coronary artery disease	0.5-0.8 cun
			Dizziness	0.5-0.8 cun
			Erysipelas (Skin infection)	0.5-0.8 cun
			Extremities pain	0.5-0.8 cun
			Floating vision	0.5-0.8 cun
			Gastritis	0.5-0.8 cun
			Heart disease	0.5-0.8 cun
			Heart issues	0.5-0.8 cun
			Hypertension	0.5-0.8 cun
			Middle finger numbness	0.5-0.8 cun
			Myocardial infarction	0.5-0.8 cun
			Myocarditis	0.5-0.8 cun
			Nasal disease	0.5-0.8 cun
			Palpitations	0.5-0.8 cun
			Paraesthesia	0.5-0.8 cun
			Pericarditis	0.5-0.8 cun
			Rheumatic fever (Esp. arthritis)	0.5-0.8 cun
			Skin infection (Erysipelas)	0.5-0.8 cun
			Stomach diseases	0.5-0.8 cun
			Stomach distension	0.5-0.8 cun
			Stomachache	0.5-0.8 cun
			TIA	0.5-0.8 cun
			Vertigo due to anemia	0.5-0.8 cun
			Vertigo: due to cerebral anemia	0.5-0.8 cun
			Arthritic pain of the fingers	0.5-0.8 cun
			Knee pain cold	0.5-0.8 cun
			Palpitations	0.5-0.8 cun

Notes:

Point	Name Pinyin	English Name	Indications	Insertion
88.03	Tong Tian	Passing Sky	Leg weakness	0.5-1.0 cun
			Acute Cardiac rheumatism	0.5-1.0 cun
			Bradicardia	0.5-1.0 cun
			Cardiac pain	0.5-1.0 cun
			Cerebral ischemia	0.5-1.0 cun
			Coronary artery disease	0.5-1.0 cun
			Dizziness	0.5-1.0 cun
			Erysipelas (Skin infection)	0.5-1.0 cun
			Extremities pain	0.5-1.0 cun
			Floating vision	0.5-1.0 cun
			Gastritis	0.5-1.0 cun
			Heart disease	0.5-1.0 cun
			Heart issues	0.5-1.0 cun
			Hypertension	0.5-1.0 cun
			Myocarditis	0.5-1.0 cun
			Palpitations	0.5-1.0 cun
			Paraesthesia	0.5-1.0 cun
			Pericarditis	0.5-1.0 cun
			Rheumatic fever (Esp. arthritis)	0.5-1.0 cun
			Skin infection (Erysipelas)	0.5-1.0 cun
			Stomachache	0.5-1.0 cun
			TIA	0.5-1.0 cun
			Vertigo: due to cerebral anemia	0.5-1.0 cun
			Knee pain cold	0.5-1.0 cun
			Abdominal pain lateral lower	0.5-1.0 cun
			Back & spine deformity	0.5-1.0 cun
			Edema	0.5-1.0 cun
			Excessive stomach acid	0.5-1.0 cun
			Leg pain cold	0.5-1.0 cun
			Palpitations	0.5-1.0 cun
			Scoliosis	0.5-1.0 cun
88.04	Jie Mei Yi	First Sister	Hysteromyoma	1.5-2.0 cun
			Shoulder pain syndrome (Any pain from shoulder to wrist & scapula)	1.5-2.0 cun
			Leucorrhea with red & white discharge	1.5-2.0 cun
			Abdominal pain	1.5-2.0 cun
			Lower abdominal pain (intestinal)	1.5-2.0 cun
			Menorrhagia (excessive menses)	1.5-2.0 cun
			Metritis (Uterine inflammation)	1.5-2.0 cun
			Pain in whole body	1.5-2.0 cun
			Peptic ulcer complications (Esp. hemorrhage)	1.5-2.0 cun
			Uterine inflammation (Metritis)	1.5-2.0 cun
			Vaginitis	1.5-2.0 cun
			Whole body pain	1.5-2.0 cun

129

Tung Acupuncture: A Quick Reference Guide

Point	Name Pinyin	English Name	Indications	Insertion
88.05	Jie Mei Er	Second Sister	Hysteromyoma	1.5-2.5 cun
			Leucorrhea with red & white discharge	1.5-2.0 cun
			Lower abdominal pain (intestinal)	1.5-2.5 cun
			Menorrhagia (excessive menses)	1.5-2.5 cun
			Metritis (Uterine inflammation)	1.5-2.5 cun
			Vaginitis	1.5-2.5 cun
			Gastric hemorrhage	1.5-2.5 cun
88.06	Jie Mei San	Third Sister	Hysteromyoma	1.5-2.5 cun
			Leucorrhea with red & white discharge	1.5-2.0 cun
			Lower abdominal pain (intestinal)	1.5-2.5 cun
			Menorrhagia (excessive menses)	1.5-2.5 cun
			Metritis (Uterine inflammation)	1.5-2.5 cun
			Gastric hemorrhage	1.5-2.5 cun
			Myoma of uterus	1.5-2.5 cun
88.07	Gan Mao Yi	1st Catch Cold	Common cold	0.8-1.5 cun
			Fever of unknown origin FUO (Infants)	0.8-1.5 cun
			Influenza	0.8-1.5 cun
88.08	Gan Mao Er	2nd Catch Cold	Common cold	0.8-1.5 cun
			Fever of unknown origin FUO (Infants)	0.8-1.5 cun
			Influenza	0.8-1.5 cun
88.09	Tong Shen	Passing Kidney	Acromion pain	0.3-0.5 cun
			Benign laryngeal tumors	0.3-0.5 cun
			Diabetes mellitus	0.3-0.5 cun
			Diabetes Oligoptyalism (Dry mouth)	0.3-0.5 cun
			Edema	0.3-0.5 cun
			Edema of the leg	0.3-0.5 cun
			Edema of the limbs Acute or chronic	0.3-0.5 cun
			Fibromylgia Due to kidney deficiency	0.3-0.5 cun
			Galacturia	0.3-0.5 cun
			Impotence	0.3-0.5 cun
			Kidney diseases	0.3-0.5 cun
			Laryngitis	0.3-0.5 cun
			Leucorrhea	0.3-0.5 cun
			Lumbago	0.3-0.5 cun
			Nephritis	0.3-0.5 cun
			Obesity (For slimming effect)	0.3-0.5 cun
			Oligoptyalism (Dry mouth) (DM)	0.3-0.5 cun
			Pain of the acromion	0.3-0.5 cun
			Premature ejaculation	0.3-0.5 cun
			Renal inflammation	0.3-0.5 cun
			Shoulder & back pain	0.3-0.5 cun
			Strangury	0.3-0.5 cun
			Uterine pain	0.3-0.5 cun
			Water retention	0.3-0.5 cun

Notes:

130

© **Theodore L. Zombolas PhD (AM), LAc, Dipl.Ac. (NCCAOM).** ©

Point	Name Pinyin	English Name	Indications	Insertion
88.10	Tong Wei	Passing Stomach	Abdominal pain lateral lower	0.3-0.8 cun
			Acromion pain	0.3-0.8 cun
			Back pain	0.3-0.8 cun
			Benign laryngeal tumors	0.3-0.8 cun
			Diabetes mellitus	0.3-0.8 cun
			Edema	0.3-0.8 cun
			Edema of the leg	0.3-0.8 cun
			Edema of the limbs Acute or chronic	0.3-0.8 cun
			Excessive stomach acid	0.3-0.8 cun
			Fibromylgia Due to kidney deficiency	0.3-0.8 cun
			Galacturia	0.3-0.8 cun
			Impotence	0.3-0.8 cun
			Kidney diseases	0.3-0.8 cun
			Laryngitis	0.3-0.8 cun
			Leg pain cold	0.3-0.8 cun
			Leucorrhea	0.3-0.8 cun
			Lumbago	0.3-0.8 cun
			Nephritis	0.3-0.8 cun
			Obesity (For slimming effect)	0.3-0.8 cun
			Oligoptyalism (Dry mouth) (DM)	0.3-0.8 cun
			Pain of the acromion	0.3-0.8 cun
			Premature ejaculation	0.3-0.8 cun
			Renal inflammation	0.3-0.8 cun
			Shoulder & back pain	0.3-0.8 cun
			Strangury	0.3-0.8 cun
			Uterine pain	0.3-0.8 cun

Notes:

Point	Name Pinyin	English Name	Indications	Insertion
88.11	Tong Bei	Passing Back	Acromion pain	0.5-1.0 cun
			Adhesive capsulitis	0.5-1.0 cun
			Back ache	0.5-1.0 cun
			Back pain	0.5-1.0 cun
			Benign laryngeal tumors	0.5-1.0 cun
			Biceps tendonitis	0.5-1.0 cun
			Diabetes mellitus	0.5-1.0 cun
			Edema	0.5-1.0 cun
			Edema of the leg	0.5-1.0 cun
			Fibromylgia Due to kidney deficiency	0.5-1.0 cun
			Frozen shoulder	0.5-1.0 cun
			Galacturia	0.5-1.0 cun
			Impotence	0.5-1.0 cun
			Kidney diseases	0.5-1.0 cun
			Laryngitis	0.5-1.0 cun
			Leucorrhea	0.5-1.0 cun
			Lumbago	0.5-1.0 cun
			Nephritis	0.5-1.0 cun
			Obesity (For slimming effect)	0.5-1.0 cun
			Oligoptyalism (Dry mouth) (DM)	0.5-1.0 cun
			Pain of the acromion	0.5-1.0 cun
			Premature ejaculation	0.5-1.0 cun
			Renal inflammation	0.5-1.0 cun
			Shoulder & back pain	0.5-1.0 cun
			Shoulder pain syndrome (Any pain from shoulder to wrist & scapula)	0.5-1.0 cun
			Strangury	0.5-1.0 cun
			Uterine pain	0.5-1.0 cun

Notes:

132

Point	Name Pinyin	English Name	Indications	Insertion
88.12	Ming Huang	Bright Yellow	Aplastic anemia	1.5-2.5 cun
			Back & spine deformity	1.5-2.5 cun
			Back tenderness	1.5-2.5 cun
			Blurred vision	1.5-2.5 cun
			Bone swelling (RA, OA, trauma induced)	1.5-2.5 cun
			Cholecystitis	1.5-2.5 cun
			Chorea (CNS problem) (Parkinsonism)	1.5-2.5 cun
			Chronic diseases	1.5-2.5 cun
			Chronic fatigue (Liver deficiency) Chorea	1.5-2.5 cun
			Cirhossis	1.5-2.5 cun
			Double vision (Strabismus)	1.5-2.5 cun
			Dry eyes	1.5-2.5 cun
			Erythropenia	1.5-2.5 cun
			Eye dryness	1.5-2.5 cun
			Hepatitis	1.5-2.5 cun
			Hepatitis A	1.5-2.5 cun
			Hepatitis chronic with jaundice	1.5-2.5 cun
			Hyper-Leucocytosis	1.5-2.5 cun
			Indigestion	1.5-2.5 cun
			Jaundice	1.5-2.5 cun
			Leukemia (Increased WBC)	1.5-2.5 cun
			Liver diseases	1.5-2.5 cun
			Liver GB diseases	1.5-2.5 cun
			Multiple sclerosis	1.5-2.5 cun
			Nocturnal shock (Nightmares)	1.5-2.5 cun
			Obesity	1.5-2.5 cun
			Ophthalmalgia	1.5-2.5 cun
			Parkinson's disease	1.5-2.5 cun
			Sciatica Due to bone spurs	1.5-2.5 cun
			Scoliosis	1.5-2.5 cun
			Spinal vertebrae spur	1.5-2.5 cun
			Spondylitis	1.5-2.5 cun
			Strabismus (Double vision).	1.5-2.5 cun
			Tinnitus	1.5-2.5 cun
			Wrist pain	1.5-2.5 cun

Notes:

133

Point	Name Pinyin	English Name	Indications	Insertion
88.13	Tian Huang	Heavenly Yellow	Aplastic anemia	1.5-2.5 cun
			Back tenderness	1.5-2.5 cun
			Blurred vision	1.5-2.5 cun
			Bone swelling (RA, OA, trauma induced)	1.5-2.5 cun
			Cholecystitis	1.5-2.5 cun
			Chorea (CNS problem) (Parkinsonism)	1.5-2.5 cun
			Chronic fatigue (Liver deficiency) Chorea	1.5-2.5 cun
			Cirhossis	1.5-2.5 cun
			Dysuria	1.5-2.5 cun
			Erythropenia	1.5-2.5 cun
			Hepatitis	1.5-2.5 cun
			Hepatitis A	1.5-2.5 cun
			Hepatitis chronic with jaundice	1.5-2.5 cun
			Hyper-Leucocytosis	1.5-2.5 cun
			Indigestion	1.5-2.5 cun
			Jaundice	1.5-2.5 cun
			Leukemia (Increased WBC)	1.5-2.5 cun
			Liver cirrhosis	1.5-2.5 cun
			Liver diseases	1.5-2.5 cun
			Liver GB diseases	1.5-2.5 cun
			Multiple sclerosis	1.5-2.5 cun
			Nocturnal shock (Nightmares)	1.5-2.5 cun
			Ophthalmalgia	1.5-2.5 cun
			Parkinson's disease	1.5-2.5 cun
			Spondylitis	1.5-2.5 cun

Notes:

134

Point	Name Pinyin	English Name	Indications	Insertion
88.14	Qi Huang	This Yellow	Aplastic anemia	1.5-2.0 cun
			Back & spine deformity	1.5-2.0 cun
			Blurred vision	1.5-2.0 cun
			Bone swelling (RA, OA, trauma induced)	1.5-2.0 cun
			Cholecystitis	1.5-2.0 cun
			Chorea (CNS problem) (Parkinsonism)	1.5-2.0 cun
			Chronic fatigue (Liver deficiency) Chorea	1.5-2.0 cun
			Cirhossis	1.5-2.0 cun
			Erythropenia	1.5-2.0 cun
			Heel pain	1.5-2.0 cun
			Hepatitis	1.5-2.0 cun
			Hepatitis A	1.5-2.0 cun
			Hepatitis chronic with jaundice	1.5-2.0 cun
			Hyper-Leucocytosis	1.5-2.0 cun
			Indigestion	1.5-2.0 cun
			Jaundice	1.5-2.0 cun
			Leucopenia	1.5-2.0 cun
			Leukemia (Increased WBC)	1.5-2.0 cun
			Liver cirrhosis	1.5-2.0 cun
			Liver diseases	1.5-2.0 cun
			Liver GB diseases	1.5-2.0 cun
			Multiple sclerosis	1.5-2.0 cun
			Nocturnal shock (Nightmares)	1.5-2.0 cun
			Ophthalmalgia	1.5-2.0 cun
			Osteoarthritis	1.5-2.0 cun
			Parkinson's disease	1.5-2.0 cun
			Scoliosis	1.5-2.0 cun
			Spinal pain	1.5-2.0 cun
			Spondylitis	1.5-2.0 cun
88.15	Huo Zhi	Fire Branch	Back pain	1.5-2.0 cun
			Blurred vision	1.5-2.0 cun
			Cholecystitis	1.5-2.0 cun
			Dizziness	1.5-2.0 cun
			Heel pain	1.5-2.0 cun
			Hepatitis A	1.5-2.0 cun
			Jaundice Which induces dizziness	1.5-2.0 cun
			Lumbago	1.5-2.0 cun
			Spinal pain	1.5-2.0 cun
88.16	Huo Quan	Fire Complete	Back pain	1.5-2.0 cun
			Blurred vision	1.5-2.0 cun
			Cholecystitis	1.5-2.0 cun
			Dizziness	1.5-2.0 cun
			Heel pain	1.5-2.0 cun
			Hepatitis A	1.5-2.0 cun
			Jaundice which induces dizziness	1.5-2.0 cun
			Lumbago	1.5-2.0 cun
			Spinal pain	1.5-2.0 cun

Tung Acupuncture: A Quick Reference Guide

Point	Name Pinyin	English Name	Indications	Insertion
88.17	Zi Ma Zhong	Center 4 Horses	Abdominal pain lateral lower	0.8-2.5 cun
			Acne	0.8-2.5 cun
			Allergic rhinitis	0.8-2.5 cun
			Allergies	0.8-2.5 cun
			Allergy, nasal	0.8-2.5 cun
			Asthma	0.8-2.5 cun
			Back ache	0.8-2.5 cun
			Back pain	0.8-2.5 cun
			Back tenderness	0.8-2.5 cun
			Breast pain	0.8-2.5 cun
			Chest & abdomen pain (Lateral)	0.8-2.5 cun
			Chest & back pain	0.8-2.5 cun
			Chest injury (Impact trauma)	0.8-2.5 cun
			Chest stuffiness	0.8-2.5 cun
			Conjunctivitis	0.8-2.5 cun
			Costalgia	0.8-2.5 cun
			Dryness of the nose	0.8-2.5 cun
			Ear pain (Middle ear infect)	0.8-2.5 cun
			Earache	0.8-2.5 cun
			Exopthalmos (Due to thyortoxicosis)	0.8-2.5 cun
			Eyes, difficulty opening (Myasthenia)	0.8-2.5 cun
			Facial nerve palsy	0.8-2.5 cun
			Facial paralysis	0.8-2.5 cun
			Facial spasm	0.8-2.5 cun
			Hearing loss	0.8-2.5 cun
			Hemiplegia	0.8-2.5 cun
			Intercostal neuralgia	0.8-2.5 cun
			Leg numbness	0.8-2.5 cun
			Loss of hearing	0.8-2.5 cun
			Lower extremity sprain/strain.	0.8-2.5 cun
			Lumbago d/t lung deficiency	0.8-2.5 cun
			Lung deficiency	0.8-2.5 cun
			Lung diseases	0.8-2.5 cun
			Myasthenia: Eyes, difficulty opening	0.8-2.5 cun
			Nasal allergy	0.8-2.5 cun
			Nasal diseases all types	0.8-2.5 cun
			Nose dryness	0.8-2.5 cun
			Pleurisy	0.8-2.5 cun
			Pleuritis	0.8-2.5 cun
			Pollen allergies	0.8-2.5 cun
			Pruritis (Itching)	0.8-2.5 cun
			Psoriasis	0.8-2.5 cun
			Pulmonary tuberculosis	0.8-2.5 cun.
			Rhinitis	0.8-2.5 cun
			Sciatica	0.8-2.5 cun
			Sciatica Due to lung deficiency	0.8-2.5 cun
			Sinusitis	0.8-2.5 cun
			Skin conditions	0.8-2.5 cun
			Skin diseases	0.8-2.5 cun
			Skin snsitiveness	0.8-2.5 cun

Tung Acupuncture: A Quick Reference Guide

Point	Name Pinyin	English Name	Indications	Insertion
			Spleen strengthen supplement Qi	0.8-2.5 cun
88.17	Zi Ma Zhong	Center 4 Horses	Teburculosis	0.8-2.5 cun
			Tinnitus	0.8-2.5 cun
			Urticaria	0.8-2.5 cun
88.18	Zi Ma Shang	Upper 4 Horses	Abdominal pain lateral lower	0.8-2.5 cun
			Acne	0.8-2.5 cun
			Allergic rhinitis	0.8-2.5 cun
			Allergies	0.8-2.5 cun
			Allergy, nasal	0.8-2.5 cun
			Asthma	0.8-2.5 cun
			Back ache	0.8-2.5 cun
			Back pain	0.8-2.5 cun
			Back tenderness	0.8-2.5 cun
			Breast pain	0.8-2.5 cun
			Chest & abdomen pain (Lateral)	0.8-2.5 cun
			Chest & back pain	0.8-2.5 cun
			Chest injury (Impact trauma)	0.8-2.5 cun
			Chest stuffiness	0.8-2.5 cun
			Chronic fatigue (Thyroid issues)	0.8-2.5 cun
			Conjunctivitis	0.8-2.5 cun
			Costalgia	0.8-2.5 cun
			Dryness of the nose	0.8-2.5 cun
			Earache	0.8-2.5 cun
			Exopthalmos (Due to thyortoxicosis)	0.8-2.5 cun
			Eyes, difficulty opening (Myasthenia)	0.8-2.5 cun
			Facial nerve palsy	0.8-2.5 cun
			Facial paralysis	0.8-2.5 cun
			Facial spasm	0.8-2.5 cun
			Hearing loss	0.8-2.5 cun
			Hemiplegia	0.8-2.5 cun
			Intercostal neuralgia	0.8-2.5 cun
			Leg numbness	0.8-2.5 cun
			Loss of hearing	0.8-2.5 cun
			Lower extremity sprain/strain.	0.8-2.5 cun
			Lumbago d/t lung deficiency	0.8-2.5 cun
			Lung deficiency	0.8-2.5 cun
			Lung diseases	0.8-2.5 cun
			Myasthenia: Eyes, difficulty opening	0.8-2.5 cun
			Nasal allergy	0.8-2.5 cun
			Nasal diseases all types	0.8-2.5 cun
			Nose dryness	0.8-2.5 cun
			Pleurisy	0.8-2.5 cun
			Pleuritis	0.8-2.5 cun
			Pollen allergies	0.8-2.5 cun
			Pruritis (Itching)	0.8-2.5 cun
			Psoriasis	0.8-2.5 cun
			Pulmonary tuberculosis	0.8-2.5 cun
			Rhinitis	0.8-2.5 cun
			Sciatica	0.8-2.5 cun
			Sciatica Due to lung deficiency	0.8-2.5 cun
			Sinusitis	0.8-2.5 cun

137

auto immune conditions

© **Theodore L. Zombolas PhD (AM), LAc, Dipl.Ac. (NCCAOM).** ©

Point	Name Pinyin	English Name	Indications	Insertion
88.18	Zi Ma Shang	Upper 4 Horses	Skin conditions	0.8-2.5 cun
			Skin diseases	0.8-2.5 cun
			Skin snsitiveness	0.8-2.5 cun
			Smoking cessation	0.8-2.5 cun
			Spleen strengthen supplement Qi	0.8-2.5 cun
			Stop smoking	0.8-2.5 cun
			Teburculosis	0.8-2.5 cun
			Tinnitus	0.8-2.5 cun
			Urticaria	0.8-2.5 cun
88.19	Zi Ma Xia	Lower 4 Horses	Abdominal pain lateral lower	0.8-2.5 cun
			Acne	0.8-2.5 cun
			Allergic rhinitis	0.8-2.5 cun
			Allergies	0.8-2.5 cun
			Allergy, nasal	0.8-2.5 cun
			Asthma	0.8-2.5 cun
			Back ache	0.8-2.5 cun
			Back pain	0.8-2.5 cun
			Back tenderness	0.8-2.5 cun
			Breast pain	0.8-2.5 cun
			Chest & abdomen pain (Lateral)	0.8-2.5 cun
			Chest & back pain	0.8-2.5 cun
			Chest injury (Impact trauma)	0.8-2.5 cun
			Chest stuffiness	0.8-2.5 cun
			Conjunctivitis	0.8-2.5 cun
			Costalgia	0.8-2.5 cun
			Dryness of the nose	0.8-2.5 cun
			Earache	0.8-2.5 cun
			Exopthalmos (Due to thyortoxicosis)	0.8-2.5 cun
			Eyes, difficulty opening (Myasthenia)	0.8-2.5 cun
			Facial nerve palsy	0.8-2.5 cun
			Facial paralysis	0.8-2.5 cun
			Facial spasm	0.8-2.5 cun
			Hearing loss	0.8-2.5 cun
			Hemiplegia	0.8-2.5 cun
			Intercostal neuralgia	0.8-2.5 cun
			Leg numbness	0.8-2.5 cun
			Loss of hearing	0.8-2.5 cun
			Lower extremity sprain/strain.	0.8-2.5 cun
			Lumbago d/t lung deficiency	0.8-2.5 cun
			Lung deficiency	0.8-2.5 cun
			Lung diseases	0.8-2.5 cun
			Myasthenia: Eyes, difficulty opening	0.8-2.5 cun
			Nasal allergy	0.8-2.5 cun
			Nasal diseases all types	0.8-2.5 cun
			Nose dryness	0.8-2.5 cun
			Pleurisy	0.8-2.5 cun
			Pleuritis	0.8-2.5 cun
			Pollen allergies	0.8-2.5 cun
			Pruritis (Itching)	0.8-2.5 cun
			Psoriasis	0.8-2.5 cun
			Pulmonary tuberculosis	0.8-2.5 cun

Point	Name Pinyin	English Name	Indications	Insertion
88.19	Zi Ma Xia	Lower 4 Horses	Rhinitis	0.8-2.5 cun
			Sciatica	0.8-2.5 cun
			Sciatica Due to lung deficiency	0.8-2.5 cun
			Sinusitis	0.8-2.5 cun
			Skin conditions	0.8-2.5 cun
			Skin diseases	0.8-2.5 cun
			Skin snsitiveness	0.8-2.5 cun
			Spleen strengthen supplement Qi	0.8-2.5 cun
			Teburculosis	0.8-2.5 cun
			Tinnitus	0.8-2.5 cun
			Urticaria	0.8-2.5 cun
88.20	Xia Quan	Lower Fountain	Bells palsy	0.3-0.5 cun
			Eye twitching	0.3-0.5 cun
88.21	Zhong Quan	Middle Fountain	Bells palsy	1.0-1.5 cun
			Eye twitching	1.0-1.5 cun
88.22	Shang Quan	Upper Fountain	Bells palsy	1.0-1.5 cun
			Eye twitching	1.0-1.5 cun
88.23	Jin Qian Xia	Lower Gold Front	Dyspepsia (Indigestion)	0.3-0.5 cun
			Epilepsy (Bilateral) (Aquired or congenital)	0.3-0.5 cun
			Headache	0.3-0.5 cun
			Skin allergy	0.3-0.5 cun
88.24	Jin Qian Shang	Upper Gold Front	Dyspepsia (Indigestion)	0.5-1.0 cun
			Epilepsy (Bilateral) (Aquired or congenital)	0.5-1.0 cun
			Headache	0.5-1.0 cun
			Skin allergy	0.5-1.0 cun

Notes:

139

Point	Name Pinyin	English Name	Indications	Insertion
88.25	Zhong Jiu Li	Middle 9 Miles	Acromion pain	0.8-2.0 cun
			Arm pain (Upper)	0.8-2.0 cun
			Cervical spondylosis	0.8-2.0 cun
			Cholecystitis	0.8-2.0 cun
			Difficult miscellaneous disease	0.8-2.0 cun
			Dizziness	0.8-2.0 cun
			Elbow joint pain	0.8-2.0 cun
			Facial spasm	0.8-2.0 cun
			Foot pain	0.8-2.0 cun
			Headache: Migraines	0.8-2.0 cun
			Hemiplegia	0.8-2.0 cun
			Insomnia	0.8-2.0 cun
			Knee pain	0.8-2.0 cun
			Leg pain cold	0.8-2.0 cun
			Migraine	0.8-2.0 cun
			Needle shock	0.8-2.0 cun
			Pain along Shaoyang channel	0.8-2.0 cun
			Pain of the acromion	0.8-2.0 cun
			Pain of the thigh	0.8-2.0 cun
			Shoulder pain	0.8-2.0 cun
			Shoulder-hand syndrome	0.8-2.0 cun
			Spinal vertebra tenderness	0.8-2.0 cun
			Spinal vertebrae spur	0.8-2.0 cun
			Spondylosis cervical	0.8-2.0 cun
			Thigh pain	0.8-2.0 cun
			Tic douroureaux	0.8-2.0 cun
			Tinnitus	0.8-2.0 cun
			Trigeminal neuralgia (tic douloureaux)	0.8-2.0 cun
			Urticaria	0.8-2.5 cun
			Urticaria on lower part of the body	0.8-2.0 cun

Notes:

140

Point	Name Pinyin	English Name	Indications	Insertion
88.26	Shang Jiu Li	Upper 9 Miles	Abdominal distension (flatulence)	0.8-2.0 cun
			Acromion pain	0.8-2.0 cun
			Arm pain	0.8-2.0 cun
			Arm pain (Upper)	0.8-2.0 cun
			Cholecystitis	0.8-2.0 cun
			Finger numbness	0.8-2.0 cun
			Flatulence	0.8-2.0 cun
			Foot pain	0.8-2.0 cun
			Hemiplegia	0.8-2.0 cun
			Insomnia	0.8-2.0 cun
			Leg pain cold	0.8-2.0 cun
			Pain of the acromion	0.8-2.0 cun
			Pain of the thigh	0.8-2.0 cun
			Parkinson's disease	0.8-2.0 cun
			Shoulder pain	0.8-2.0 cun
			Shoulder-hand syndrome	0.8-2.0 cun
			Spinal vertebra tenderness	0.8-2.0 cun
			Spinal vertebrae spur	0.8-2.0 cun
			Thigh pain	0.8-2.0 cun
			Urticaria	0.8-2.5 cun
			Urticaria on lower part of the body	0.8-2.0 cun
88.27	Xia Jiu Li	Lower 9 Miles	Acromion pain	0.8-2.0 cun
			Arm pain (Upper)	0.8-2.0 cun
			Back pain	0.8-2.0 cun
			Cholecystitis	0.8-2.0 cun
			Finger numbness	0.8-2.0 cun
			Foot pain	0.8-2.0 cun
			Hemiplegia	0.8-2.0 cun
			Insomnia	0.8-2.0 cun
			Leg pain (Anterior Tibia, shin plints, compartment syndrome)	0.8-2.0 cun
			Leg pain (Due to ischemia)	0.8-2.0 cun
			Leg pain cold	0.8-2.0 cun
			Pain of the acromion	0.8-2.0 cun
			Pain of the thigh	0.8-2.0 cun
			Parkinson's disease	0.8-2.0 cun
			Shoulder pain	0.8-2.0 cun
			Spinal vertebra tenderness	0.8-2.0 cun
			Spinal vertebrae spur	0.8-2.0 cun
			Thigh pain	0.8-2.0 cun
			Urticaria	0.8-2.5 cun
			Urticaria on lower part of the body	0.8-2.0 cun
88.28	Jie	Release Point	Chest injury (Impact trauma)	0.3-0.5 cun
			Fainting during acupuncture	0.3-0.5 cun
			Hypodermic injection pain	0.3-0.5 cun
			Qi & Blood disorders	0.3-0.5 cun
			Syncope, iatrogenic	0.3-0.5 cun
			Traumatic injury pain	0.3-0.5 cun

Tung Acupuncture: A Quick Reference Guide

Point	Name Pinyin	English Name	Indications	Insertion
88.29	Nei Tong Guan	Inner Passing Gate	CVA	1.0 cun
			Hemiplegia	1.0 cun
			Palpitations	1.0 cun
			TIA	1.0 cun
88.30	Nei Tong Shan	Inner Passing Mountain	CVA	1.0 cun
			Hemiplegia	1.0 cun
			Palpitations	1.0 cun
			TIA	1.0 cun
88.31	Nei Tong Tian	Inner Passing Sky	CVA	1.0 cun
			Hemiplegia	1.0 cun
			TIA	1.0 cun
			Palpitations	1.0 cun
88.32	Shi Yin	Voice Loss	Aphasia	1.0-1.5 cun
			Aphonia	1.0-1.5 cun
			Hoarseness (Loss of voice)	1.0-1.5 cun
			Loss of voice due to stroke	1.0-1.5 cun
			Parathyroiditis	1.0-1.5 cun
			Thyroid tumor	1.0-1.5 cun
			Thyroiditis	1.0-1.5 cun
			Tonsillitis	1.0-1.5 cun
99.01	Er Huan	Ear Ring	Alcohol intoxication (Esp. hangover)	0.2 cun
			Hangover	0.2 cun
			Nausea & vomiting	0.2 cun
99.02	Mu Er	Wood Ear	Gonorrhea	0.2 cun
			Hepatalgia (Liver pain)	0.2 cun
			Hepatomegaly	0.2 cun
			Liver cirrhosis	Just touch cartilage
99.03	Huo Er	Fire Ear	Dyspnoea, palpitations	0.2 cun
			Extremities pain	0.2 cun
			Knee pain	0.2 cun
			Knee pain	0.2 cun
			Palpitations	0.2 cun
			Thigh pain	0.2 cun
99.04	Tu Er	Earth Ear	Diabetes mellitus	0.2 cun
			Erythrocytosis (Increased RBC)	0.2 cun
			High fever	0.2 cun
			Hyperemia (High fever)	0.2 cun
			Hysteria	0.2 cun
			Nervousness	0.2 cun
			Neurosis	0.2 cun
99.05	Jin Er	Gold Ear	Allergic rhinitis	0.2 cun
			Sciatica	0.2 cun
			Scoliosis (Esp. abnormal lumbar curve)	0.2 cun
			Scoliosis	0.2 cun
99.06	Shui Er	Water Ear	Astigmatism	0.2 cun
			Dry mouth	0.2 cun
			Lumbago	0.2 cun
			Myopia (Short sightedness)	0.2 cun

142

Tung Acupuncture: A Quick Reference Guide

Point	Name Pinyin	English Name	Indications	Insertion
99.07	Er Bei	Back of Ear	Blurred vision	Micro-puncture
			Laryngitis	Micro-puncture
			Vision blurred	Micro-puncture
			Vocal cord nodules & polyps	Micro-puncture
99.08	Er San	Ear Three	Common cold	Micro-puncture
			Diarrhea	Micro-puncture
			Migraine	Micro-puncture
1010.01	Zheng Hui	Uprightness Meeting	Aphasia	0.1-0.3 cun
			Cerebral palsy	0.1-0.3 cun
			Chronic pain (Any type)	0.1-0.3 cun
			Cloudiness thinking and fatigue (Neurasthenia)	0.1-0.3 cun
			Coccyx pain	0.1-0.3 cun
			Coma	0.1-0.3 cun
			Facial nerve palsy	0.1-0.3 cun
			Hemiplegia	0.1-0.3 cun
			Pain chronic (Any type)	0.1-0.3 cun
			Parkinson's syndrome	0.1-0.3 cun
			Parkinsonism	0.1-0.3 cun
			Phantom pain	0.1-0.3 cun
			Seizure in children	0.1-0.3 cun
			Stress	0.1-0.3 cun
			Stroke	0.1-0.3 cun
			Tics	0.1-0.3 cun
			Weakness general	0.1-0.3 cun
1010.02	Zhou Yuan	Prefecture Round	Asthma	0.1-0.3 cun
			Hemiplegia	0.1-0.3 cun
			Lumbago	0.1-0.3 cun
			Sciatica	0.1-0.3 cun
			Weakness general	0.1-0.3 cun
1010.03	Zhou Kun	Prefecture Elder Brother	Asthma	0.1-0.3 cun
			Brain tumor	0.1-0.3 cun
			Hemiplegia	0.1-0.3 cun
			Lumbago	0.1-0.3 cun
			Sciatica	0.1-0.3 cun
			Weakness general	0.1-0.3 cun
1010.04	Zhou Lun	Prefecture Mountain	Asthma	0.1-0.3 cun
			Benign brain tumors	0.1-0.3 cun
			Brain tumor	0.1-0.3 cun
			Hemiplegia	0.1-0.3 cun
			Lumbago	0.1-0.3 cun
			Sciatica	0.1-0.3 cun
			Weakness general	0.1-0.3 cun

143

© Theodore L. Zombolas PhD (AM), LAc, Dipl.Ac. (NCCAOM). ©

Tung Acupuncture: A Quick Reference Guide

Point	Name Pinyin	English Name	Indications	Insertion
1010.05	Qian Hui	Anterior Meeting	Coma	0.1-0.3 cun
			Dizziness	0.1-0.3 cun
			Faintness (Syncope)	0.1-0.3 cun
			Headache tension (Frontal to temporal)	0.1-0.3 cun
			Nervousness (Psychoneurosis)	0.1-0.3 cun
			Parkinson's disease	0.1-0.3 cun
			Parkinson's syndrome	0.1-0.3 cun
			Shock (Esp. neurogenic type)	0.1-0.3 cun
1010.06	Hou Hui	Posterior Meetings	Coccyx pain	0.1-0.3 cun
			Coma	0.1-0.3 cun
			Compartment syndrome	0.1-0.3 cun
			CVA	0.1-0.3 cun
			Dizziness	0.1-0.3 cun
			Entrapment neuropathy	0.1-0.3 cun
			Heel pain	0.1-0.3 cun
			Hemiplegia	0.1-0.3 cun
			Pain in the heel	0.1-0.3 cun
			Parkinson's disease	0.1-0.3 cun
			Scoliosis	0.1-0.3 cun
			Spinal pain (Esp. thoracic lumbar)	0.1-0.3 cun
1010.07	Zong Shu	Total Pivot	Aphasia	Micro-puncture
			Cholera	0.1-0.2 cun
			Disphagia Due to stroke	0.1-0.2 cun
			Neck pain	0.1-0.2 cun
			Palpitations	0.1-0.2 cun
			Regurgitation	Micro-puncture
			Stroke with aphasia	Micro-punture
			Tongue rigidity (Aphasia due to apoplexy)	0.1-0.2 cun
			Vomiting	0.1-0.2 cun
1010.08	Zhen Jing	Tranquility	Cloudiness thinking and fatigue (Neurasthenia)	0.1-0.2 cun
			Hysteria	0.1-0.2 cun
			Insomnia	0.1-0.2 cun
			Leg weakness	0.1-0.2 cun
			Nocturnal crying (Child)	0.1-0.2 cun
			Pain chronic (Any type)	0.1-0.2 cun
			Phantom pain	0.1-0.2 cun
			Tremor (Due to anxiety, endocrine & MS)	0.1-0.2 cun
1010.09	Shang Li	Upper Mile	Blurred vision	0.1-0.2 cun
			Headache	0.1-0.2 cun
1010.10	Si Fu Er	4 Bowels 2nd	Abdominal distension (flatulence)	0.1-0.2 cun
			Blurred vision	0.1-0.2 cun
			Headache	0.1-0.2 cun
1010.11	Si Fu Yi	4 Bowels 1st	Abdominal distension	0.1-0.2 cun
			Blurred vision	0.1-0.2 cun
			Headache	0.1-0.2 cun
1010.12	Zheng Ben	Upright Source	Common cold (Feverish conditions)	Micro-puncture
			Psychosis (Paranoid type)	0.1-0.2 cun
			Rhinitis allergic	0.1-0.2 cun

Point	Name Pinyin	English Name	Indications	Insertion
1010.13	Ma Jin Shui	Horse Gold Water	Back ache radiating to lower limb	0.1-0.3 cun
			Bladder stones	0.1-0.3 cun
			Chest pain	0.1-0.3 cun
			Kidney stones	0.1-0.3 cun
			Low back pain	0.1-0.3 cun
			Lower back pain due to Kidney deficiency	0.1-0.3 cun
			Lumbago	0.1-0.3 cun
			Lumbar sprain (Acute)	0.1-0.3 cun
			Nephritis	0.1-0.3 cun
			Nephrolithiasis (Kidney stone)	0.1-0.3 cun
			Renal calculus Acute & chronic	0.1-0.3 cun
			Renal colic	0.1-0.3 cun
			Rhinitis	0.1-0.3 cun
1010.14	Ma Kuai Shui	Horse Fast Water	Bladder stones	0.1-0.3 cun
			Cystitis	0.1-0.3 cun
			Cystolithiasis	0.1-0.3 cun
			Frequent urination	0.1-0.3 cun
			Galacturia	0.1-0.3 cun
			Lower back pain due to Kidney deficiency	0.1-0.3 cun
			Polyuria	0.1-0.3 cun
			Rhinitis	0.1-0.3 cun
			Spinal pain	0.1-0.3 cun
			Urinary bladder stone	0.1-0.3 cun
			Urination difficulty	0.1-0.3 cun
			Urination frequent	0.1-0.3 cun
1010.15	Fu Kuai	Bowels Ease	Abdominal distension	0.1-0.3 cun
			Abdominal pain	0.1-0.3 cun
			Hernia	0.1-0.3 cun
1010.16	Liu Kuai	Six Fastness	Bladder stones	0.1-0.2 cun
			Frequent painful urination	0.1-0.2 cun
			Ureterolith (Uriter stone)	0.1-0.2 cun
			Urethritis	0.1-0.2 cun
			Urithral calculus	0.1-0.2 cun
1010.17	Qi Kuai	Seven Fastness	Bladder stones	0.5-1.5 cun
			Facial nerve palsy	0.5-1.5 cun
			Frequent painful urination	0.5-1.5 cun
			Ureterolith (Uriter stone)	0.5-1.5 cun
			Urithral calculus	0.5-1.5 cun
			Weakness general	0.5-1.5 cun
1010.18	Mu Zhi	Wood Branch	Cholecystitis	0.1-0.3 cun
			Cholilithiasis	0.1-0.3 cun
			Gall stone	0.1-0.3 cun
			Hysteria	0.1-0.3 cun
			Leg weakness	0.1-0.3 cun
			Parkinson's syndrome	0.1-0.3 cun

Notes:

145

© **Theodore L. Zombolas PhD (AM), LAc, Dipl.Ac. (NCCAOM).** ©

Point	Name Pinyin	English Name	Indications	Insertion
1010.19	Shui Tong	Water Through	Asthma	0.1-0.5 cun
			Asthmatic breathing	0.1-0.5 cun
			Blurred vision	0.1-0.5 cun
			Bronchitis	0.1-0.5 cun
			Bronchitis (Chronic)	0.1-0.5 cun
			Chronic fatigue Due to kidney deficiency	0.1-0.5 cun
			Cough	0.1-0.5 cun
			Cough & asthma	0.1-0.5 cun
			Dizziness	0.1-0.5 cun
			Dyspnoea	0.1-0.5 cun
			Fatigue	0.1-0.5 cun
			Fibromyalgia Due to kidney deficiency	0.1-0.5 cun
			Hemiplegia due to K deficiency	0.1-0.5 cun
			Hiccup	0.1-0.5 cun
			Low back sprain/strain d/t Qi blockage	0.1-0.5 cun
			Lower back pain	0.1-0.5 cun
			Lower back pain due to Kidney deficiency	0.1-0.5 cun
			Lumbar sprain (Acute)	0.1-0.5 cun
			Lung diseases	0.1-0.5 cun
			Shen-K'uei syndrome (For males)	0.1-0.5 cun
			Thigh pain and soreness	0.1-0.5 cun
			Tongue rigidity (Aphasia due to apoplexy)	0.1-0.5 cun
			Vertigo	0.1-0.5 cun
			Vomiting	0.1-0.5 cun
1010.20	Shui Jin	Water Gold	Aphasia due to apoplexy	0.1-0.1 cun
			Asthma	0.1-0.5 cun
			Asthmatic breathing	0.1-0.5 cun
			Blurred vision	0.1-0.5 cun
			Bronchitis	0.1-0.5 cun
			Bronchitis (Chronic)	0.1-0.5 cun
			Chronic fatigue Due to kidney deficiency	0.1-0.5 cun
			Cough	0.1-0.5 cun
			Cough & asthma	0.1-0.5 cun
			Dizziness	0.1-0.5 cun
			Dyspnoea	0.1-0.5 cun
			Fatigue	0.1-0.5 cun
			Fibromyalgia Due to kidney deficiency	0.1-0.5 cun
			Hemiplegia due to K deficiency	0.1-0.5 cun
			Hiccup	0.1-0.5 cun
			Low back sprain/strain d/t Qi blockage	0.1-0.5 cun
			Lower back pain	0.1-0.5 cun
			Lower back pain due to Kidney deficiency	0.1-0.5 cun
			Lung diseases	0.1-0.5 cun
			Shen'K'uei syndrome	0.1-0.5 cun
			Thigh pain and soreness	0.1-0.5 cun
			Tongue rigidity (Aphasia due to apoplexy)	0.1-0.5 cun
			Vertigo	0.1-0.5 cun
			Vomiting	0.1-0.5 cun

Point	Name Pinyin	English Name	Indications	Insertion
1010.21	Yu Huo	Jade Fire	Extremities pain (Hands & feet)	0.1-0.3 cun
			Knee pain	0.1-0.3 cun
			Maxilla pain	0.1-0.3 cun
			Sciatica	0.1-0.3 cun
			Shoulder pain	0.1-0.3 cun
1010.22	Bi Yi	Nasal Wing	Back sorness	0.1-0.2 cun
			Extremities pain (Hands & feet)	0.1-0.2 cun
			Facial nerve palsy	0.1-0.2 cun
			Fatigue	0.1-0.2 cun
			Hemiplegia	0.1-0.2 cun
			Loin sorness	0.1-0.2 cun
			Migraine	0.1-0.2 cun
			Pharyngitis	0.1-0.2 cun
			Sciatica	0.1-0.2 cun
			Scoliosis	0.1-0.2 cun
			Speaking trouble	0.1-0.2 cun
			Supra orbital pain	0.1-0.2 cun
			Tongue pain (heat related)	0.1-0.2 cun
			Vertigo	0.1-0.2 cun
			Whole body pain	0.1-0.2 cun
1010.23	Zhou Huo	Prefect Fire	Low back pain	0.1-0.3 cun
			Lumbago	0.1-0.3 cun
			Palpitations	0.1-0.3 cun
			Rheumatism	0.1-0.3 cun
			Tiredness	0.1-0.3 cun
1010.24	Zhou Jin	Prefect Gold	Lumbago	0.1-0.3 cun
			Rheumatism	0.1-0.3 cun
			Sciatica	0.1-0.3 cun
1010.25	Zhou Shui	Prefect Water	Extremities weakness	0.1-0.3 cun
			Paralysis Lower limb	0.1-0.3 cun
			Spinal pain	0.1-0.3 cun
1010.26	Ti Shen	Raise The Spirits	Exhaustion	0.1-0.2 cun
			Fatigue	0.1-0.2 cun
1010.27	Du Zong	Supervising Chief	Governing vessel pain	Micro-puncture
DT01	Fen Chi Shang	Upper Separation Branch	Armpit odor	1.0-1.5 cun
			Bromhidrosis	1.0-1.5 cun
			Diabetes Mellitus	1.0-1.5 cun
			Drug poisoning (Mild case)	1.0-1.5 cun
			Food poisoning	1.0-1.5 cun
			Gas poisoning (CO)	1.0-1.5 cun
			Gonorrhea	1.0-1.5 cun
			Halitosis	1.0-1.5 cun
			Pruritis	1.0-1.5 cun
			Scabies	1.0-1.5 cun

Tung Acupuncture: A Quick Reference Guide

Point	Name Pinyin	English Name	Indications	Insertion
DT02	Fen Chi Sha	Lower Separation Branch	Gonorrhea	0.5-1.0 cun
			Armpit odor	0.5-1.0 cun
			Bromhidrosis	0.5-1.0 cun
			Diabetes Mellitus	0.5-1.0 cun
			Drug poisoning (Mild case)	0.5-1.0 cun
			Food poisoning	0.5-1.0 cun
			Gas poisoning (CO)	0.5-1.0 cun
			Halitosis	0.5-1.0 cun
			Mastitis	0.5-1.0 cun
			Pruritis	0.5-1.0 cun
			Scabies	0.5-1.0 cun
DT03	Chi Shing	Seven Stars	Common cold children	Micro-puncture
			Headache due to common cold	Micro-puncture
			High fever in children	Micro-puncture
			Vomiting	Micro-puncture
DT04	Wu Ling	5 Mountain Ranges	Athrosclerosis	Micro-puncture
			Blurred vision Due to hypertension	Micro-puncture
			Coma	Micro-puncture
			Common cold	Micro-puncture
			Fever	Micro-puncture
			Fever high	Micro-puncture
			Headache	Micro-puncture
			Headache acute	Micro-puncture
			Hemianesthesia	Micro-puncture
			Hemiplegia	Micro-puncture
			Hypertension	Micro-puncture
			Lumbago	Micro-puncture
			Stomachache acute	Micro-puncture
			Stroke parlysis of extremities	Micro-puncture
			Vertigo: hypotensive	Micro-puncture
			Vision blurred due to hypertension	Micro-puncture
			Vomiting	Micro-puncture
DT05	Shuang Feng	Double Phoenix	Ateriosclerosis	Micro-puncture
			Cervical bone spurs with hand numbness	Micro-puncture
			Finger numbness	Micro-puncture
			Leg numbness	Micro-puncture
			Leg pain cold	Micro-puncture
			Numbness in extremites	Micro-puncture
			Pain in extremities	Micro-puncture
			Toe numbness	Micro-puncture
DT06	Chiu Hou	9 Monkeys	Coronary artery disease	Micro-puncture
DT07	San Jin	Three Gold	Knee joint pain	Micro-puncture
			Knee pain	Micro-puncture
			Knee pain anterior	Micro-puncture
			Knee pain cold	Micro-puncture
			Knee pain cold (Bone spur or chronic condition)	Micro-puncture

Tung Acupuncture: A Quick Reference Guide

Point	Name Pinyin	English Name	Indications	Insertion
DT08	Jing Zhi	Essence Branch	Foot soreness Difficulty walking	Micro-puncture
			Leg pain (Sorness & distending pain)	Micro-puncture
			Leg pain	Micro-puncture
			Leg swelling	Micro-puncture
			Pain of legs	Micro-puncture
DT09	Jin Lin	Gold Forest	Arteriosclerosis	Micro-puncture
			Pain of the thigh	Micro-puncture
			Sciatica	Micro-puncture
			Thigh pain	Micro-puncture
			Thigh pain and soreness	Micro-puncture
DT10	Ting Chu	Top Pillar	Chest pain	Micro-puncture
			Lumbago	Micro-puncture
			Lumbago acute	Micro-puncture
DT11	Hou Shin	Behind Heart	Furunculosis	Micro-puncture
			Gastritis chronic	Micro-puncture
			Hemiplegia	Micro-puncture
			Myocardial infarction acute	Micro-puncture
DT12	Kan Mao San	3rd Catch Cold	Common cold	Micro-puncture
DT15	San Chiang	Three Rivers	Amenorrhea	Micro-puncture
			Enteritis acute	Micro-puncture
			Lumbago	Micro-puncture
			Uteritis	Micro-puncture
DT16	Huang Ho	Paired Rivers	Arm pain	Micro-puncture
			Elbow tennis	Micro-puncture
			Shoulder pain	Micro-puncture
			Tennis elbow	Micro-puncture
DT17	Chong Xiao	Expanding Heaven	Dizziness	Micro-puncture
			Headache	Micro-puncture
			Headache: Occipital	Micro-puncture
			Neck pain	Micro-puncture
VT01	Huo O Chiu	Throat Moth 9	Sore throat	Micro-puncture
			Throat itching	Micro-puncture
			Thyroiditis	Micro-puncture
			Tracheal obstruction	Micro-puncture
VT02	Shi Er Hou	12 Monkeyes	Asthma adult	Micro-puncture
			Common cold	Micro-puncture
			Typhoid fever	Micro-puncture
VT03	King Wu	Gold Five	Costalgia (Rib pain)	Micro-puncture
			Dyspnoea	Micro-puncture
			Indigestion	Micro-puncture
			Rib pain (costaglia)	Micro-puncture
VT04	Wei Mao Chi	Stomach Hair 7	Enteritis	Micro-puncture
			Gastric hemorrhage	Micro-puncture
			Palpitations	Micro-puncture
			Stomach disease	Micro-puncture
VT05	Fu Chao 23	Bowel Nest 23	Colic abdominal pain	Micro-puncture
			Enteritis	Micro-puncture
			Nephritis	Micro-puncture
			Periumbilical pain	Micro-puncture
			Uteritis	Micro-puncture
VT06	Chun Ma	Lip Numbness	Lip numbness	0.5 cun

Tung Acupuncture: A Quick Reference Guide

Point	Name Pinyin	English Name	Indications	Insertion
Ear	Apex		Bells palsy	Micro-puncture
			Common cold	Micro-puncture
			Conjunctivitis (Redness of the eyes)	Micro-puncture
			Eye diseases	Micro-puncture
			Facial paralysis	Micro-puncture
			Glaucoma	Micro-puncture
			Hidrosis	Micro-puncture
			Insomnia	Micro-puncture
			Keratitis	Micro-puncture
			Myocarditis	Micro-puncture
			Oral ulceration	Micro-puncture
			Palpitations	Micro-puncture
			Skin diseases	Micro-puncture
			Stye	Micro-puncture
			Sublingual swelling	Micro-puncture
			Tachycardia	Micro-puncture
Ear	Back		Acne	Micro-puncture
			Mandible pain (Difficulty opening mouth)	Micro-puncture
			Psoriasis	Micro-puncture
			Urticaria	Micro-puncture
Ear	Tip		Alcohol intoxication	Micro-puncture
			Hypertension	Micro-puncture
			Skin snsitiveness	Micro-puncture
L1	Shui Chung	Water Center	Constipation	0.8-1.0 cun
			Kidney disease	0.8-1.0 cun
			Menstruation irregular	0.8-1.0 cun
			Nephritis	0.8-1.0 cun
			Spinal pain	0.8-1.0 cun
			Thirst	0.8-1.0 cun
L2	Shui Fu	Water Bowels	Constipation	0.8-1.0 cun
			Cystolithiasis	0.8-1.0 cun
			Diabetes mellitus	0.8-1.0 cun
			Dysuria	0.8-1.0 cun
			Ejaculation early	0.8-1.0 cun
			Enteritis	0.8-1.0 cun
			Headache	0.8-1.0 cun
			Impotence	0.8-1.0 cun
			Insomnia	0.8-1.0 cun
			Kidney disease	0.8-1.0 cun
			Lumbago	0.8-1.0 cun
			Nephritis	0.8-1.0 cun
			Nephritis acute	0.8-1.0 cun
			Thirst	0.8-1.0 cun

150

Tung Acupuncture

Points Not To Be Used On Pregnant Patients

Points not to be used on pregnant patients

22.04	55.01	66.03	77.17
22.05		66.04	77.19
		66.10	77.20
		66.11	77.21
		66.12	

Notes:

Notes:

Tung Acupuncture

Micro-Puncture

Micro-Puncture:

Micro-puncture is an important element of classical acupuncture treatment. The ancient Chinese archive of medicine, the Su-Wen mentions that sharp stone blades originated in the Eastern China. The practice of phlebotomy, or bloodletting, also dates back to ancient times. Hippocrates, "the father of modern medicine," first advocated bloodletting in ancient Greece as a method of bringing an unbalanced, diseased person back to equilibrium. This technique was also done in Egyptian times and earlier as well. Today the term "phlebotomy" refers to the act of drawing blood for laboratory study or blood transfusion.

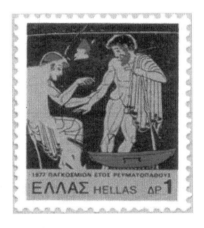

Ancient Greek painting on a stamp, showing a physician bleeding a patient.

Bloodletting was a common practice in early America. Unfortunately, America's first president, George Washington, is said to have had a total of 80 ounces of his blood drained from his body over a series of bleedings in a short period of time. With such a large amount of blood removed, Washington failed to improve, and died from hypovolemia the evening of December 14, 1799.

In recent history, modern allopathic medicine has returned to the use of bleeding patients. With the advent of microsurgery, the use of leeches in medicine, known as hirudotherapy, made its comeback in the 1980's. This medicinal use of leeches to drain off stagnant blood dates back to the beginnings of civilization.

There is also a practice called therapeutic phlebotomy which refers to the drawing of blood in specific cases of an increased amount of red blood cells in the body, like hemochromatosis, polycythemia. This is done to reduce the amount of circulating red blood cells, thus reducing the risk of blood clots, which can lead to pulmonary embolus, stroke and even death.

157

Tung Acupuncture: A Quick Reference Guide

Most acupuncturists believe that the purpose of bloodletting is to remove the stagnancy/sluggishness of the Qi and/or Blood in the body. Therefore micro-puncture is believed to enhance blood circulation and stop related pain. In fact, clinical research reveals that blood letting has effects such as detoxification, sedation, anti-emetic, anti-inflammation, prevents congestion, stops itching, and diarrhea and can be used in a life saving emergency. Further study shows micro-puncture can change blood composition, regulate body temperature, activate the immune system, accelerate digestion and in some instances produce full recovery after an encounter of trauma to the central nervous system (CNS).

Tung's acupuncturists would therefore prefer to use micro-puncture wherever they find that the patient's clinical condition requires a speedier recovery. There are several similarities in the methods used when comparing Tung's with the descriptions such as those in the ancient archives of the Yellow Emperor of Internal Medicine. I have found Tung's style of micro puncture to be much easier to apply.

The tools used to practice Tung's style micro-puncture are simple and effective. It was only after the Chinese civil war, when Master Tung joined the army and moved to Taiwan in 1949, that he began to improve his specially designed triangular needles using stainless steel instead. His 3 inch-long needles are nowhere to be found now except those kept by some of his old students.

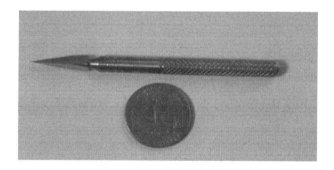

Hand made three edged needle similar to the one used by Master Tung

Master Tung would not use commercially available bleeding needles, such as plum-flower needles, Spring Punchers (popular in Japan), or the cheap machine-made needles produced in Taiwan and Mainland China, as he found them to be clinically inadequate.

158

Tung Acupuncture: A Quick Reference Guide

The needle used today is called a three-edged needle, which was developed from the Sharp needle of the Nine Needles created in the ancient times.

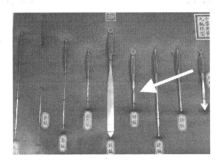

Today's three-edged needle is made of stainless steel, with a length of approximately 6 cm. It is produced with a round handle, which tapers to a sharp tip incorporating three blades in a triangular head. There are different size blades available on the market.

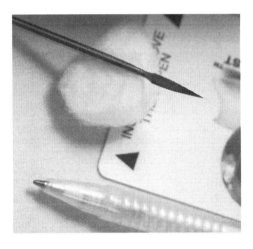

Typical Three-Edged needle of today.

Micro-puncture is often used to treat different kinds of disorders, such as the excess syndrome, heat syndrome, dispel blood stasis, obstruction of meridians and pain due to blockage. It acts to resuscitate, purge fire and subside swellings, relieve pain, loss of consciousness, sore throat, local congestion or swelling and so on.

It is imperative that a detailed history is taken, on your patient as predisposing medical conditions may lead to severe complications once bled. Bleeding should never be performed on someone taking any blood thinning medication such as Warfarin (Coumadin) nor have any clinical blood coagulation disorders, as these patients will have difficulty stopping any bleeding. Diabetic patients and patients with cardiac disorders should not be blood let. Anemic or weak and lethargic patients usually do not require blood-letting, but it should not be ruled out but for a very small group of patients.

Other instruments can be used for bleeding such as the different types of lancets available to diabetics used for blood glucose testing. We will focus on the three-edged needle for the purpose of our discussion.

Most classical acupuncturist bleed the distal veins, this practice should be done with great caution and care, as one may find it difficult to stop the bleeding or have problems controlling the bleeding afterwards. In some cases, common micro-puncture sites are restricted to existing acupuncture points, like GV 26, UB 40, and LU 5. As well, some practitioners will bleed painful symptomatic areas, as well as bleed small superficial arteriole supplied areas. Medically trained practitioners or properly trained acupuncturists who are very familiar with anatomy would never risk puncturing potentially dangerous anatomic structures.

Tung style micro-puncture differs from the other methods as its practitioners look for areas with the most capillary dilatation and disease referral area for bleeding purposes. These guidelines make Tung's method more effective than the Western veinosection, and alternative style puncture/cupping technique. In fact, both of these bleeding methods can remove up to 100-200cc blood from the patient. Tung's practitioners consider such an amount extreme for an already compromised patient to bear. From either a hemodynamic or classical Eastern Medical teaching point of view. A large quantity of Micro-puncturing is considered not only unnecessary but also possibly fatal. The outcome must always dictate the treatment.

Today's practitioners should know that micro-puncture or blood letting is suitable for both acute as well as chronic illness. Tung's Orthodox acupuncture protocol usually applies micro puncture on a weekly basis, releasing only a few drops of blood each time. Besides bleeding any founded capillary dilation sites, Tung's acupuncture followers may puncture points such as 1.26 Chin-Wu for treating delayed healing and chronic abscess, 7.10 Tz'u-Hua-Fu for acute gastritis or myocardium infarction, 9.07 Erh-Pei for acute tonsillitis, DT 07 San-King for arthritic acute or chronic knee pain. 10.12 Cheng-Pen for allergic rhinitis or acute manic depression psychoses.

Tung Acupuncture: A Quick Reference Guide

The basic requirements for performing micro-puncture procedures are:

A. First review the patient's medical history to confirm the presence or absence of any blood related diseases. Look for any medical condition that would be adversely affected with the micro puncture procedure. Proper protection and protocol should be adhered to, especially in the event of such conditions such as HIV, Hepatitis virus and the like.

   Hepatitis A = may be transmitted via blood. Incubation 15-45 days.
   Hepatitis B = major blood born pathogen. Incubation 50-180 days.
   Hepatitis C = major blood born pathogen. Incubation 20-90 days.
   HIV = major blood born pathogen. Incubation 2-15 years.

B. One should strictly follow basic procedures for maintaining a clean treatment field including adequate preparation of the micro-puncture site.

C. You should have all supplies ready and available close by during the procedure. This includes:

   a. Disinfectant such as tincture of iodine or hydrogen peroxide.
   b. 70% isopropyl alcohol.
   c. Cotton balls or gauze sponges.
   d. Bleeding needle.
   e. Sharps bottle
   f. Band-aids
   g. Protective gloves

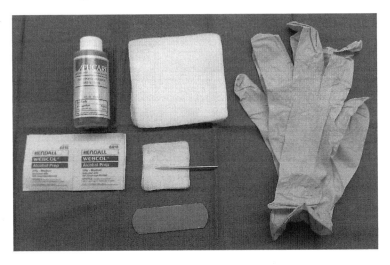

One can see from the above supplies, that micro-puncture does not involve additional supplies other than what should be available in the clinic.

161

Tung Acupuncture: A Quick Reference Guide

Step one:
Place the patient in a comfortable position. Keep in mind this position is for both the patient and practitioner. It is important to maintain a healthy and stable posture during this procedure.

Step two:
Locate the micro-puncture site that will be used. Make an indentation with your fingernail. This makes the area of the skin numb; it also helps to accurately locate the spot with the bleeding needle.

Step three:
Prepare the micro-puncture site with clean technique. First use a disinfectant solution of iodine or hydrogen peroxide to clean the skin. Then wipe the site with isopropyl alcohol. The technique that should be used is a circular motion, starting from the center and working outwards, away from the puncture site. This ensures that you wash away from the site, thus not contaminating the puncture site with a wiping back and forth motion from outside to inside.

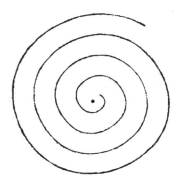

Step four:
The needle should be held firmly in the hand between the index finger and the thumb. The middle finger is used as a stop, which is positioned on the needle at a level of how far you wish to puncture. This will control and prevent the needle from piercing deeper than preferred.

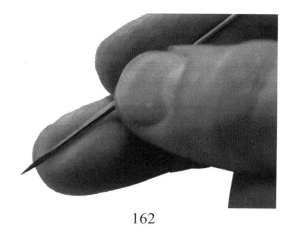

162

Step five:

Position your needling hand on the patient next to the puncture site, and secure the area with your other hand. Remember to keep from contaminating the site.

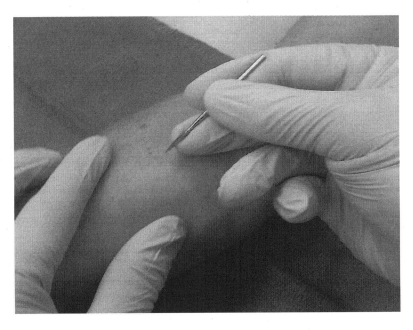

Step six:

The needling is done with a twisting motion of the wrist. It is imperative that the puncturing is done in one swift movement. This will reduce the discomfort the patient may experience.

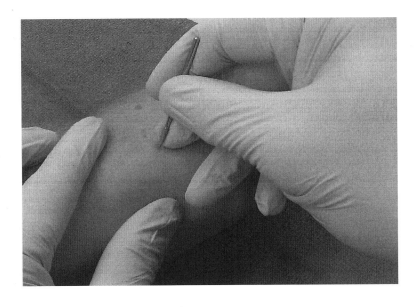

163

Step seven:
Once the needle is withdrawn, discard the needle in the sharps container. Begin to squeeze out small amounts of blood. If needed continue squeezing for more blood.

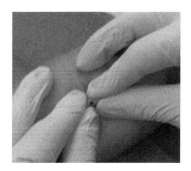 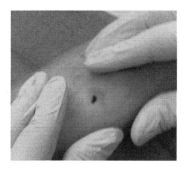

Notice in the picture, the site of bleeding was not located on a vessel, but on an area of capillary dilatation. This necessitates the need for squeezing to remove blood.

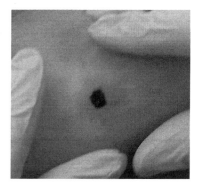

Step eight:
Once all the required blood has been removed, it is essential that a proper dressing be applied. Band-aids are adequate, unless excessive unexpected bleeding occurs. In this case, apply pressure long enough to stop any and all bleeding. Then apply a dressing appropriately. If proper technique is followed, there is no need for the use of antibiotics afterwards.

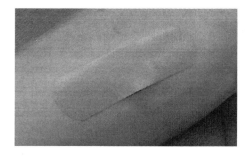

It is important to note that the needle is three-edged. This has the inherent result of having the puncture site remain open, as the skin contracts. If a straight edge instrument were to be used, the skin would naturally close on itself. For this reason it is advisable that the patient refrain from getting the puncture site wet for a period up to one week. This is to prevent any possibility of infection as the wound heals. It may be necessary to apply antibiotic ointment later on in the healing process if warranted. This antibiotic ointment can be purchased over the counter at local drug stores.

Bleeding sites tend to be local, as opposed to needling which is done distal to the area of injury. There are a number of bleeding sites in Tung style acupuncture that are used which are located distal to the area of injury, these can be used to enhance the healing process of the patient.

Notes:

Tung Acupuncture: A Quick Reference Guide

Theodore L. Zombolas PhD (AM), LAc, Dipl.Ac. (NCCAOM)

Ted has been involved in the Oriental arts since the age of 13 when he began his martial arts training. He has since studied and taught various styles of oriental fighting systems such as Karate, Gung Fu, Ju-Jitsu, Escrema and Jeet Kune Do. Along with these studies, Ted was introduced into the world of Oriental healing arts. His exposure to herbal remedies, which are used for treating injuries sustained in training and combat, opened him to the world of Traditional Chinese Medicine.

He has been certified as an Emergency Medical Technician, Respiratory Therapist, Cardiovascular Perfusionist and Acupuncturist. Ted began his studies in TCM in the United States, and completed his studies in Acupuncture at the Chinese Medicine and Acupuncture Academy of Toronto (CMAAT), and is now certified by the National Certification Commission of Acupuncture and Oriental Medicne (NCCAOM). Ted also holds a diploma from the International Medical Acupuncture Training Program from Beijing China, and has also completed an extensive internship at the Yunnan Provincial Hospital of Traditional Chinese Medicine, Kunming China. With Ted's continued hunger for knowledge and studies, he has earned a PhD in Alternative Medicine, and continues to learn healing methods from around the world.

He was first introduced to Tung style acupuncture in 2004 through an acquaintance, and was so impressed with the results it obtained, that he did some research into this amazing style and found Dr. Carson. In August 2009 he achieved Advanced Level in Tung's Orthodox Acupuncture in the World Tung Acupuncture Association (WTAA) under Dr. Carson. Ted has been instrumental in organizing and hosting WTAA classes, which has allowed many more acupuncturists to learn and benefit from this remarkable family style of acupuncture.

Ted has lectured on Traditional Chinese Medicine in China, Canada and the United States, and is the author of *"Food as Medicine A Traditional Chinese Medical Perspective"*. Ted has published numerous articles on western cardiovascular medicine, and he has also written a paper on his unique technique on smoking cessation, which has become a standard with many acupuncturists around the world.

Ted's style of acupuncture includes Tung's Orthodox Acupuncture, Balance Method Acupuncture and Traditional Chinese Acupuncture. He incorporates food as medicine along with herbal medicinals in his practice, including Tai Qi and Qi Gong. He is also a practitioner of Dit Da style medicine, specializing in traumatology and athletic enhancement.

167